AIDS TRANSMISSION
Challenges in the New Millennium

AIDS TRANSMISSION
Challenges in the New Millennium

Editor
G.C. Satpathy

KALPAZ

Published by

Kalpaz Publications
C-30, Satyawati Nagar,
Delhi – 110052
Ph.: 011-47034999, 9811692060
www.kalpazpublications.com
E-mail: kalpaz@hotmail.com

Distribution Network
gyanbooks.com
India, USA, Canada, UK, Australia, France

ISBN: 978-93-5722-488-8 (PB)

First Published, 2024

Printed at: Gyan Press, Delhi.

Aids Transmission: Challenges in the New Millennium
Editor: G.C. Satpathy

Preface

A decade after the Human Immunodeficiency Virus (HIV) was first identified as the cause of Acquired Immune Deficiency Syndrome (AIDS), the disease has been reported in nearly all developing and industrial countries. In many developing countries the HIV/AIDS epidemic is spreading rapidly. Because AIDS kills mostly prime-age adults, it increases the number of children who lose one or both parents; some of these orphans suffer permanent consequences, due to poor nutrition or withdrawal from school. Numbers cannot begin to capture the suffering caused by the disease. AIDS is not alone in causing human suffering, however especially in the developing world.

HIV/AIDS is a fatal, sexually transmitted disease (STD). After an initial week or two of flu-like symptoms, the disease has no visible effects on the infected person during an asymptomatic period, which can be as short as two years or as long as 20. Although the average time without symptoms is about ten years in industrial countries, limited data suggest that it might be as short as five years among the poorest people in the poorest countries. Like other STDs, HIV/AIDS is difficult to transmit except by sex or other direct contact with the bodily fluids of an infected person. The major modes of transmission are sexual intercourse, reuse of contaminated syringes by injecting drug users, infection via birth or nursing from mother to child, reuse of needles in medical settings and transfusions of contaminated blood or blood products.

HIV/AIDS is a large and growing problem and that governments can and should actively confront the epidemic. Some policies will be much more effective than others and it distinguishes between activities that can be undertaken by households and the private sector, including non-governmental organisations (NGOs); those that should be initiated by developing country governments; and those that should be most strongly supported by donor governments and the international development community.

This book presents a comprehensive accessible account of HIV/AIDS, its emergence, transmission, challenges raised by it, and preventive methods. It will prove informative and ideal reference tool for all the concerned.

Editor

Contents

1

Introduction

The acquired immune deficiency syndrome (AIDS), is a large and growing problem and that today's society is facing. The human immunodeficiency virus (HIV) is a fatal, among the sexually transmitted diseases (STD). After an initial week or two of flulike symptoms, the disease has no visible effects on the infected person during an asymptomatic period, which can be as short as two years or as long as 20. Although the average time without symptoms is about ten years in industrial countries, limited data suggest that it might be as short as five years among the poorest people in the poorest countries. Then, in all but a very small proportion of cases, the disease destroys the immune system. This leaves the infected person vulnerable to other infectious diseases, which are typically fatal within six to 24 months.

Like other STDs, HIV is difficult to transmit except by sex or other direct contact with the bodily fluids of an infected person. The major modes of transmission are sexual intercourse, reuse of contaminated syringes by injecting drug users, infection via birth or nursing from mother to child, reuse of needles in medical settings and transfusions of contaminated blood or blood products. About three-quarters of HIV transmission worldwide is through sex. Of these sexual transmissions, about three- quarters involve heterosexual intercourse and one-quarter involve sexual relations between men.

In developing countries, sex accounts for an even greater proportion of cases. In sub-Saharan Africa, Asia and the Caribbean, sexual transmission is overwhelmingly between men and women; less than 1 per cent involve homosexual acts. In Latin America and Eastern Europe, however, sex between men still accounted for most sexual transmission as recently as the early 1990s.

Another most important means of transmission after sexual intercourse is the sharing of unsterilised needles among injecting drug users. Transmission through injecting drug use has been the primary mode of transmission in China and Southeast Asia, except in Thailand, where heterosexual transmission has outpaced transmission by needle sharing.

Injecting drug use is also thought to account for about one-quarter to one-third of transmissions in Brazil and Argentina. HIV can spread through a population of injecting drug users extremely rapidly, in some locales infecting the majority within a few months.

The importance of mother-to-child transmission varies widely across countries. The major mode of infection among infants can occur in the uterus through contact with the mother's blood at birth or later through breastfeeding. Since mother-to-child transmission can occur only if the mother is herself infected, it is most common in widespread heterosexual epidemics, such as in sub-Saharan Africa.

HIV may also be spread through medical injections. In some of the poorest countries, injections are the preferred delivery system for a variety of medications and the same syringe may be used on many people in one day without sterilisation between injections.

However, even in these countries, medical injections with dirty needles are thought to account for less than 5 per cent of all HIV infections. Transmission through blood transfusions, once a cause for concern in many countries, has been nearly eliminated in many high and middle-income countries by routine screening of blood for transfusions.

In developing countries, transmission through the blood supply has yet to be eliminated, especially where HIV prevalence rates are high among blood donors and where screening blood for HIV has not yet become routine.

But while transmission through transfused blood and other blood products greatly increases the risk of medical care and can rapidly spread HIV among specific populations, HIV transmission through transfusions has never accounted for more than about 10 per cent of total HIV infections, even in developing countries.

One of the most obvious impact of AIDS is on the expectancy and health. Measuring and predicting these impacts are difficult, not only because of the lack of quality data, but also because the relative size of an impact depends on many factors besides the spread of AIDS, including success in fighting other health problems. Available evidence discussed below suggests that in the most severely affected countries, AIDS threatens to reverse a century of progress in the fight against infectious diseases. Elsewhere, it is likely to account for an increased share of the infectious disease burden. Even so, AIDS is only one of many health problems confronting people in developing countries.

Indeed, the poorer the country, the more likely it is that other problems—including easily treated problems like malnutrition and diarrhoea—account for a large share of the burden of disease. The proportion of total deaths caused by a disease is an imperfect representation of its burden on society because it ignores illness and does not distinguish among the deaths of people of different ages.

Murray and Lopez have estimated the cost of diseases in terms of disability-adjusted life years, or DALYs. Introduced by the World Development Report 1993, a DALY includes the disability as well as the mortality effects of disease and uses age weights to discount the importance of infant and elderly deaths.

In 1990, poor health resulted in the loss of about 265 DALYs per thousand persons per year in developing countries, almost twice the 124 DALYs per thousand per year lost in industrial countries. Since HIV/AIDS deaths entail substantial disability before death and disproportionally strike prime-age adults, HIV/AIDS has a larger impact on health measured as DALYs than when measured as a share of total deaths.

However, the difference is not large: Murray and Lopez project that HIV/AIDS would account for almost 3 per cent of all DALYs lost in developing countries in the year 2020, up from 0.8 per cent in 1990. One reason that HIV/AIDS does not account for a larger percentage of lost DALYs is that other causes of death in developing countries also entail substantial disability and premature death. When we focus attention on infectious disease, the contribution of HIV/AIDS to the disease burden looms larger. Such a focus is particularly relevant to our overarching purpose of identifying the appropriate roles for developing country governments in the fight against AIDS because economic theory, public health teaching and long-standing practice all affirm that governments should play a significant role in preventing the spread of infectious disease.

By 2020 infectious diseases, which currently account for about 30 per cent of deaths and one-quarter of lost DALYs in developing countries, will have declined to about 14 per cent of both measures. But the contribution of HIV/AIDS to the infectious disease burden in developing countries is projected to increase sharply, from about 2 per cent of deaths and 3 per cent of lost DALYs to about 14 per cent of deaths and nearly one-fifth of lost DALYs. Moreover, because HIV is an increasingly important factor in the spread of TB, it is estimated that about one out of four TB deaths among HIV-negative people in 2020 would not have occurred in the absence of the HIV epidemic.

In many developing countries the HIV/AIDS epidemic is spreading rapidly. In major cities of Argentina, Brazil, Cambodia, India and Thailand, more than 2 per cent of pregnant women now carry HIV. These levels are similar to those found ten years ago in such African countries as Zambia and Malawi, where more than one in four pregnant women are now infected. Meanwhile, the disease is spreading rapidly in Asia.

In Latin American and the Caribbean countries the number of new infections has been steady at about 200,000 per year for several years, while the countries of eastern Europe and central Asia are experiencing the initial stages of rapid spread. Only in North America and western Europe has the number of new infections declined from its peak in 1986, but even here the future of the epidemic is unclear as it invades lower-income populations whose education and access to health care more closely resemble those of the developing world.

AIDS is clearly taking an immense and growing human toll. Because AIDS kills mostly prime-age adults, it increases the number of children who lose one or both parents; some of these orphans suffer permanent consequences, due to poor nutrition or withdrawal from school. Numbers cannot begin to capture the suffering caused by the disease.

AIDS is not alone in causing human suffering, however especially in the developing world. Given the many other pressing problems, how much time, effort and resources should governments devote to fighting AIDS? Views differ widely. Some people consider AIDS to be a late-twentieth-century version of the Black Death, which devastated Europe in the fourteenth century.

According to this view, governments should do everything in their power to slow the epidemic. Others think that governments should do little or nothing, either because they think AIDS will not be a major problem in their country or because they think that governments are powerless to change the private behaviour that spreads the virus.

AIDS usually strikes prime-age adults, often people who are raising children and are at or near the peak of their income potential, because it is sexually transmitted. In the absence of AIDS, prime-age adults tend to be less vulnerable to sickness and death than children, adolescents, or old people.

Accordingly, AIDS casts an even larger shadow on the health of prime-age adults and the welfare of their dependants. In Africa, where other infectious diseases decline less quickly than in other regions and HIV/AIDS infection rates are assumed to be levelling off in many areas, HIV/AIDS will count for about one-third of these deaths

The health impacts of the disease alone are ample cause for concern. There are additional reasons why the development community in general and policymakers in particular should be concerned about the HIV/AIDS epidemic.

First, widespread poverty and unequal distribution of income that typify underdevelopment appear to stimulate the spread of HIV.

Second, the accelerated labour migration, rapid urbanisation and cultural modernisation that often accompany growth also facilitate the spread of HIV.

Third, at the household level AIDS deaths exacerbate the poverty and social inequality that are conducive to a larger epidemic, thus creating a vicious circle.

Poverty and gender inequality make a society more vulnerable to HIV. The idea that poverty and gender inequality exacerbate AIDS is supported by an exploratory analysis of national level aggregate data on HIV infection rates. When examining the influence of gender inequality on HIV infection, one must hold constant as much as possible other cultural influences which may be correlated with gender inequality across countries.

The first of these, the ratio of mates to females in urban centers, varies remarkably across countries: some countries have fewer male urban residents than female and others have 40 per cent more males. Other things being equal, one might suppose that commercial sex would be more common in cities where men greatly outnumber women and that HIV levels would therefore be higher. Cities in which men ages 20 to 39 greatly outnumber women do in fact have significantly higher HIV infection rates. For the average country, increasing the job opportunities for young women so that the ratio of mates to females in urban areas falls, for example, from 1.3 to 0.9, would decrease the HIV infection rate by about 4 percentage points. The second measure related to gender inequality included in the analysis is the gap between adult male and female literacy rates. Again, there is great variation across countries, the literacy rate among men being as much as 25 percentage points higher than among women in some countries. When women are much less literate than men, they may be less able to bargain effectively with men and thus be at greater risk in sexual encounters.

A country that improves per capita income and reduces inequality, for example, by implementing investment policies that generate jobs and raise economic growth, will reduce its risk of suffering an AIDS epidemic or help to minimize an epidemic already under way. If, in addition, the country acts to close the literacy and urban employment gaps between men and women, HIV would have even more difficulty spreading.

Unfortunately, some of the very processes that might achieve these goals can also stimulate the spread of AIDS. And other policies that sometimes accompany growth, without necessarily contributing to it, can likewise worsen the epidemic. Some studies have suggested that immigration itself contributes to economic growth. This would hardly be surprising, since immigrants are often among the hardest-working and most enterprising people in any country. However, a cross-country regression analysis suggests that countries with larger immigrant populations tend to have larger AIDS epidemics: other things being equal, a country in which 5 per cent of the population is foreign- born can expect to have an infection rate about 2 percentage points higher than a country with no foreign-born. If immigration is beneficial to economic growth, reducing immigration may slow it, a result that, in addition to many other negative effects, may stimulate the spread of AIDS.

Attempting to screen out HIV-positive immigrants is unlikely to be very effective, since immigrants are more likely to become infected after they have arrived in a new country, when they are disconnected from the social networks of their former homeland than before leaving home. Economic development projects that do not generate sufficient net economic returns after covering the cost of mitigating negative impacts, including the spread of AIDS, should be rejected as undesirable—even if the gross returns are quite large.

Sometimes a low-income society beginning rapid growth may face an increased risk of AIDS as a result of a broad shift from conservative social norms to more liberal attitudes; these attitudes often include greater individual freedom, especially for women. Controlling for all other variables described above, a high degree of social conservatism is associated to a statistically significant degree with lower rates of HIV infection. This does not necessarily imply that governments should attempt to instill or maintain social conservatism simply to minimize HIV; such broad social values may in any event be very difficult for governments to shape. However, the evidence does suggest the usefulness of an explicit government education policy that would help young people entering a rapidly modernising society to recognise and avoid risky sexual encounters. A final factor in the regression analysis that is not associated with development but can be readily affected by government policy is the level of militarisation.

Populations in badly hit countries will decline in absolute terms and that there will be an associated collapse in economic output. However, the available evidence suggests that the impact of AIDS on these variables, although varying across countries, will generally be small relative to other factors. Moreover, at a very crude level, declines in population growth due to HIV/AIDS will tend to offset declines in economic growth, so that the net impact on gross domestic product (GDP) growth per capita will generally be small.

HIV/AIDS is expected to reduce population growth rates in many countries, but in no country is an absolute decline in population expected. The latest projections suggest that declines in population growth rates from HIV/AIDS mortality will range from about 0.1 percentage point in Thailand to 2.3 percentage points in Botswana and that the median country's population growth rate will decline by about 1 percentage point.

Over time, such a reduction in growth would result in a significantly smaller population than would have existed in the absence of AIDS. In Zambia, for example, the population is predicted to be 7 per cent smaller in 2005 than it would have been without AIDS. In two countries with very severe AIDS epidemics, Botswana and Zimbabwe, the projections suggest that by 2010 the population will cease growing. The impact of AIDS on economic growth is a much more complex issue than the impact on population growth.

The inadequacy of GDP per capita as a measure of human welfare is striking when changes in per capita GDP are used to measure the impact of AIDS. Other things held constant, the death of people with higher incomes will reduce average income—even though the welfare of those who remain alive has not changed. Conversely, the death of those with lower incomes raises average income, without necessarily improving the lot of any surviving individual and despite the suffering and economic losses of the families of those who died. Further, increased spending on health care and funerals is included in GDP calculations.

As a result, per capita GDP may increase, even though overall well-being has not improved and the incomes of survivors have been reduced. With these caveats in mind, it is nonetheless possible to estimate the size of the epidemic's impact on individual incomes. This impact will depend on characteristics of the country, including the severity of the epidemic, the efficiency of the labour market, the proportion of the treatment cost of AIDS financed from savings, the distribution of HIV infection by productivity of worker, the time lost from work by the person with AIDS and others as a result of his or her sickness and the effectiveness of household and community formal and informal insurance mechanisms.

Because AIDS kills prime-age adults, many of whom are at the peak of their economic productivity, the shock of AIDS to the labour market is one mechanism through which AIDS might affect growth. However, in economies with substantial unemployment, firms should find it easy replace sick or deceased workers, particularly if they are not key personnel. Other things being equal, the impact of the AIDS epidemic will be small until the economy begins to grow and is constrained by labour supply rather than by insufficient demand. Another factor that is likely to have a significant effect on the size of the macroeconomic impact of the epidemic is the percentage of AIDS treatment costs financed from savings.

Since spending on AIDS treatment is likely to reduce the capital available for more productive investment, the higher the proportion of care financed from savings, the larger the reduction in growth resulting from the epidemic. If one takes these factors into consideration, a rough estimate would be that a generalised epidemic, would reduce per capita GDP by as much as half a percentage point per year. In some very poor sub-Saharan African countries, growth rates in GDP per capita that are already negative may deteriorate even further as a result of the AIDS epidemic.

But some countries with severe AIDS epidemics, including Botswana, Thailand and Uganda, have been growing rapidly. With per capita growth rates in excess of 5 per cent per year, a reduction of 0.5 per cent in per capita growth will not be crippling. For these countries, as for many other countries where the epidemic may peak at lower infection levels, the more serious consequences will be the impacts on public health spending and on poverty. The macroeconomic effects of AIDS are likely to be small in most countries, but, severely affected countries will experience quite large impacts on their health sector and on the poor.

The effect on the health sector will be to increase the price and reduce the availability of health care for everyone, which will tend to hurt the poor most. Furthermore, among the households that suffer an AIDS death, lower-income households will be less able than others to cope with the medical expenses and other impacts, including loss of income. One important way in which AIDS is likely to exacerbate poverty and inequality—and indeed, one of the most tragic effects of the epidemic—is the increase in the number of children who lose one or both parents. To be sure, AIDS is not the only cause of orphanhood: in some countries other causes of prime-age adult death may orphan many more children than AIDS.

For many people the human suffering caused by the epidemic is reason enough for governments to be involved. However, there are other important reasons for government involvement, some of which are not so readily evident. Analysis of these rationales for government involvement is a necessary foundation for considering how governments should confront HIV/AIDS. One economic rationale for government involvement in HIV prevention is very straightforward: prevention is much cheaper than treatment and avoids the sickness and death that are the final outcome of the disease. This argument is particularly important in the many low-income countries where governments remain committed to publicly financed curative health care.

In such countries, the high cost of AIDS treatment starkly reveals the scarcity of resources. As the number of AIDS cases and treatment costs mount, it becomes painfully evident that AIDS treatment is consuming public resources that could have been used for other human needs. Yet governments may find it very difficult to restrict financing for AIDS treatment without at the same time reassessing their commitment to publicly financed health care.

Indeed, in many countries there are political pressures to subsidise AIDS treatment at a higher level than other health care services and these pressures are likely to grow as the number of people with HIV increases.

For all these reasons, a government that wishes to continue subsidising health care should initiate aggressive prevention efforts as early in the epidemic as possible. Even governments that are attempting to reduce subsidies for curative care would do well to invest in HIV prevention, since political pressures for subsidised care may be very difficult to resist.

A government does not subsidise curative health care and that it is able to resist all pressures to do so. Given that HIV/AIDS is primarily transmitted by sex, would there still be a rationale for government intervention to reduce its spread? The answer from a public economics perspective is yes.

To understand why, it is useful to first consider the public economics rationale for government intervention against other contagious diseases, such as TB. If all markets worked perfectly, governments would not need to be involved in the fight against these diseases. Instead, each person at risk of infection would pay an appropriate share of the cost of reducing his or her risk.

There is no mechanism other than government through which individuals can pay this amount. Since a person infected with TB is likely to consider only the benefits to himself when deciding whether to pay for treatment, without government intervention people infected with TB would be cured less often than everyone else would prefer.

Economists call the benefits of treatment that are not captured by the person paying for the treatment external benefits and the negative impacts on others of not getting treatment external costs. These externalities, if large, are a strong economic justification for government intervention. In giving advice on how governments should spend scarce public resources, economists look for evidence of large externalities or public goods.

Where these exist, markets are said to have failed and public intervention to address the market failure is warranted. In the case of TB, malaria and other diseases that may strike people regardless of their individual behaviour, the public economics arguments for government intervention due to market failure are clear. At first consideration, it may appear that externalities and public goods are not a significant concern in the case of STDs, including HIV.

Since most STD transmission occurs as a result of a voluntary act between two people, each can weigh his or her risk and proceed only if the benefits of doing so outweigh the risks. The problem, of course, is that the decision of these two people has consequences for many others, endangering marital sex and procreation as well as more casual sexual relationships. In public economics terms, there are external benefits associated with refraining from risky sex.

Since an individual cannot capture these benefits, he or she will be less prudent than would otherwise be the case. The result: higher STD infection rates and a greater risk of infection for everyone who is sexually active, even those who are monogamous, since most people cannot be sure that their partner is also monogamous.

In such a situation, government intervention is justified if it can increase the incentives for the most sexually active individuals to practice safer sex (or for injecting drug users to adopt safer injecting behaviour) to the point that their decisions more closely reflect consideration for the social consequences of risky behaviour. The arguments above for government intervention to prevent the spread of STDs apply even more strongly to HIV/AIDS.

In addition to being sexually transmitted, HIV/AIDS has two characteristics that worsen the market failures associated with the disease—and suggest that governments should be particularly concerned about HIV prevention. The most obvious is that AIDS cannot be cured and is almost always fatal. Since individuals have little control over their exposure to TB and since people who have HIV and TB can spread TB even to people who are HIV-negative, the link between HIV and TB further strengthens the arguments for a government role in controlling HIV.

While this link suggests that HIV/AIDS should receive special attention, the close epidemiological relationship between HIV and other STDs, means that in practice any effective strategy against HIV will almost certainly involve stepped-up prevention efforts against other STDs and vice versa. Since the monitoring problem described above applies equally to all STDs, governments would have a role in STD control even in the absence of HIV.

Because HIV multiplies manyfold the external costs associated with a case of gonorrhoea or genital ulcer disease, the presence of HIV strengthens the argument for government intervention to control the spread of all STDs. In some countries, HIV/AIDS has now been present for two decades, long enough for most people to know that it adds a mortal risk to sexual liaisons; yet surveys show that an alarmingly large proportion of people in some countries still do not know how to protect themselves.

In other societies, the disease is still new, an invisible danger spreading through an unsuspecting citizenry that, because of HIV's two-to-twenty-year asymptomatic period, has yet to be jolted by a sudden upsurge in AIDS deaths.

In either society, only the government has the incentives and the capacity to generate the information that permits people to take the first steps toward self-protection. Information about the state of the epidemic and how to avoid infection is a true public good. Although it is possible to restrict access to information, for example, by selling it in magazines available only to subscribers, valuable information has a tendency to spread beyond those to whom it is sold. Therefore, private firms have less incentive to produce and sell information and will produce less of it than is socially desirable. This is particularly true of information from epidemiological monitoring of infection rates in various groups in society. The value of public health surveillance lies in announcing the results, so that people are aware of the disease in their midst and can take steps to protect themselves by reducing risky behaviour.

The public role in the production of new information reaches beyond monitoring the epidemic to include various types of research that enable a more effective response. In all countries, governments will require country-specific information about how to identify and reach people at highest risk of becoming infected and spreading HIV to others.

AIDS has created new human rights concerns and cast harsh new light on long-standing problems. Thus, the universally recognised obligation of governments to protect people from harm at the hands of others is a compelling reason for governments to play an important role in society's response to HIV. Because people can be infected with HIV and transmit it to others for years before they become ill, the disease defines and creates a new minority group in society. Government responses to the difficult task of balancing the interests of the infected against the interests of others have varied widely. The human rights rationale for a government role related to HIV/AIDS is dramatic and unambiguous in instances where sexual relations are compelled by force Here the government's overarching 'bility in protecting individuals from physical l forced exploitation is reinforced by the :rest in preventing the spread of HIV.

2

Emergence of the Epidemic

During early 1980s, a strange new epidemic emerged among North American homosexual men. It was first seen in the large gay communities of New York and California among young men who were very sexually active. These men became mysteriously ill with infections and tumors that, according to previous experience, were rarely serious and rarely combined in the same individual. Certainly they had never been seen in epidemic proportions in such a narrowly defined risk group. One of the infectious agents was *Pneumocystis carinii*, a usually harmless micro-organism that thrives around us and even inside of us.

Like many other organisms in our environment, *P. carinii* routinely colonizes most of us, at an early age, with no ill effects under ordinary circumstances. It could harm only severely malnourished or ill people or children, not vigorous young men. The same was generally true for Kaposi's sarcoma (KS), the tumour most often seen in the new epidemic. KS had previously been seen in aging men in the United States and Europe, but it was uncommon and rarely aggressive. It was more frequent and serious in Africa, but still no great threat.

It was soon discovered that some impairment of the immune system that normally protects us from invaders had allowed the bizarre and fatal combination of infections and tumours. The condition was marked by a rapid decline of certain blood cells, or T-helper cells, whose cell wall includes a crucial molecule known as CD_4. These CD_4-positive cells are major players in our immune system. CD_4^+ cells are essential to fight all types of invaders. In this epidemic, their impairment was apparently not inborn but somehow acquired, so the disorder came to be called AIDS: acquired immunodeficiency syndrome. The Center for Disease Control (CDC) found that those who developed AIDS had invariably had sex with someone who concurrently had AIDS or later developed the disease. Apparently it was transmitted sexually, most likely by means of seminal fluid. Then AIDS began to occur among hemophiliacs, but not by sexual transmission. Hemophilia is a congenital disease, seen only in men, in which the blood does not clot normally. It is effectively treated with transfusions of blood that contains clotting factors, but apparently blood could also transmit AIDS. This transmission route was later confirmed when AIDS appeared among intravenous drug users who had shared needles with infected gay men.

The transmission of AIDS in semen and blood, its epidemic spread, and its sudden occurrence in otherwise healthy men suggested an infectious agent, probably a virus. In 1982 or 1983, only two years into the epidemic, a likely suspect was found at the Institute Pasteur of Paris by Franqoise Barre-Sinoussi, Jean-Claude Chermann, Luc Montagnier, and colleagues. The new virus was discovered in an enlarged lymph node taken from a young homosexual man. He had not yet developed AIDS, but AIDS patients were found to have the same virus in their blood.

In 1984, American researchers Mika Popovic, Bob Gallo, and colleagues showed that most AIDS patients had this virus, while a control group of healthy subjects did not. Meanwhile, the virus infected three lab workers who later developed AIDS. As far as most scientists were concerned, this tragedy supplied the last piece of the puzzle. According to a reasoning process based on Koch's postulates, an agent is linked to a disease in four steps.

First, the agent is observed in every case of the disease.

Second, it is isolated from people with the disease, then grown in pure culture.

Third, the culture causes the disease when inoculated into susceptible subjects (in this case, the unfortunate lab workers).

Fourth, the agent is observed and recovered from the experimentally infected subjects.

But these researchers identified the new virus, and the Gallo team grew the virus to high levels of infectivity, 'enabling rapid production of kits to diagnose the infection. The virus was soon known as HIV: human immunodeficiency virus. Perhaps no other virus in history has become so widely known in so short a time. CD_4 does not exist solely to give passage to HIV. It did not evolve to serve as the HIV receptor. In fact, its main job is sentry duty: it recognizes intruders and arouses various fighter cells against them. In an ironic twist, HIV uses this guardian molecule to enter and ultimately destroy the cells that carry it on their surface.

For survival, HIV defends by attacking: it cripples the immune system that would destroy or control it. Its effects are slow to show because, up to a point, the cells it destroys can be replenished. But eventually its steady killing reduces the quantity and quality of CD_4^+ cells, causing immunodeficiency. By the time people have full-blown AIDS, they cannot cope with invading organisms that normal people accommodate or fight off every day. The organisms that threaten AIDS patients are not only invaders from our external environment but insiders like *P. carinii.* These members of our internal ecosystem—our natural flora—are usually kept in their place by many factors, including a healthy immune system. But given the opportunity to overgrow or grow in the wrong place, they can cause "opportunistic" infection. Several studies of the natural course of AIDS have shown that certain opportunistic infections always become fatal once HIV is acquired and persists in the blood and other organs of the body. Where did this treacherous and apparently new virus come from? As the Bible says, "There is no new thing under the sun." HIV may be truly new, but it is more likely an old virus that has gained a new level of virulence, enabling it to cause human immunodeficiency.

When AIDS was first seen in North America and then in Europe and Africa, epidemiologists were baffled. Most epidemics can be traced to one focal point, but this one seemed to be spreading independently on three continents. North American and European AIDS were soon regarded as one epidemic, brought to Europe from America by gay men.

Meanwhile, a different type of AIDS surfaced among a few central Africans living in Belgium and France. This disease was transmitted heterosexually, appeared mainly in women, and had come directly from Africa. Today AIDS is generally accepted to be more than one epidemic caused by a whole family of HIV types, subtypes, and strains.

The main epidemic in North America and Europe is caused by HIV type 1 (HIV-1). Now spreading fast to South America, this Western HIV is apparently becoming ever more lethal or virulent as it is passaged through the human population. That is, it gains strength each time it enters a new person, reproduces in the CD_4^+ cells, then bursts out to circulate and infect another person. This process of cycling to virulence seems to be an HIV family trait. All members of the family, including HIV-1, were probably much less deadly when they first encountered humans. They had to reach a threshold of cycles and new infections before they could cause AIDS and premature death. If so, then HIV may have been with us for millennia.

It can suddenly cause AIDS because of some change in us or in its own makeup. So far, research indicates that all members of the HIV family can cause AIDS (some faster than others)-but a very few people can block the disease. The study began with a sample of more than one thousand gay men, who were examined every three months. These subjects belonged to the subgroup known to be at highest risk for AIDS: young gay men who seek rough and anonymous sex with multiple partners. Some of the sample were HIV-infected before the study began, but they focused on those who became infected as the study proceeded. These men, who so far number about fifty, had been followed for an average of ten to twelve years.

As usual with HIV-1, each case started with acute infection. Though brief and sometimes hardly noticeable, that flu-like illness was accompanied by the generation of permanent and specific HIV antibodies. Our immune system normally greets any invader by producing specific antibodies. They remain forever on call, should the invader reappear. If it does, they are geared to recognize and tag it as an enemy to be destroyed.

HIV antibodies are evidence of seropositivity. Their appearance signifies seroconversion: the first point at which serum was found to contain the virus. The acute stage was followed by a period free of symptoms or disease, which usually lasted several years. But of those infected early in the study, more than 75 per cent had developed AIDS, and twenty-three have died. Three individuals developed the disease within only eighteen months of initial infection. At the opposite end of the spectrum, the two lucky ones shown no sign of immunodeficiency. Incidentally, their work offers further proof that HIV is the agent of AIDS.

Of the twenty-three men who died, each acquired HIV infection before development of any immune disturbance. And not a single case of AIDS-or any sign of immunodeficiency-has developed among the many hundreds of men who had remained HIV-negative over the years.

However, a few researchers still doubt HIV is the agent of AIDS. One of their arguments is that Kaposi's sarcoma has occurred, though rarely, in young gay men with no sign of immunodeficiency. Recent evidence indicates that a newly discovered virus, sexually transmissible but unrelated to HIV, may be involved in KS. And while KS can occur without HIV, it clearly runs a much more aggressive course in HIV-positive people. Based on the linear progression of AIDS development, it is found that about 95 per cent of homosexual men infected with HIV-1 will eventually develop AIDS. Their symptom-free period will vary according to a bell-shaped curve. Very few individuals will develop AIDS in the first year after infection or in the "last" year, projected to be fifteen to twenty years after infection. Most people will progress to AIDS after an average asymptomatic period of about ten years. Their two nonprogressors remain well not because of virus variation but because of host variation. In other words, these men did not get an unusually weak virus but are, for some reason, unusually well defended hosts. All of us are genetically programmed to offer a more or less effective immune response to HIV and other invaders. The response to any invader involves many factors, all of which can vary.

With HIV, an important variation is seen in the cells that carry the CD_4 molecule. From person to person, these cells are more or less hospitable to HIV access, entry, and multiplication. Their two AIDS-free subjects have maintained extremely low levels of circulating virus since their initial infection. In contrast, subjects who have developed AIDS quickly have had extremely high levels during the entire period. Naturally, we are looking hard for the precise factor that seems to protect the nonprogressors. More clues to virus and host variation can be found by comparing HIV and AIDS in the three, major risk groups: homosexual men, IV drug users, and hemophiliacs.

All three groups are susceptible to HIV-1, but they differ in their AIDS frequency rates and their length of symptom-free periods. AIDS occurs at a somewhat higher rate among gay men than among IV drug users and hemophiliacs, even though the sexual transmission of HIV is far less efficient than its transmission by injection. For IV drug users and hemo-philiacs, certain host factors are known to lower AIDS frequency and lengthen the symptom-free period. All other things being equal, the younger a hemophiliac the better his defense against AIDS. As for drug users, the frequent sharing of syringes means frequent exposure to HIV. However, once infected, they derive a small benefit from this dangerous practice. The constant injection of foreign blood seems to dull or confuse the immune response, leading to cell *anergy* (the opposite of *energy*), which slightly curbs reproduction of the CD_4^+ cells. This, in turn, slightly curbs multiplication of HIV, since the virus depends on host reproductive mechanisms. Much evidence indicates that host factors, more than virus factors, are responsible when HIV is thwarted; conversely, host factors are less responsible when the virus thrives. All HIVs seem to be viable and virulent, and some have found ways to increase their damage. So HIV needs no help from a weak defense, but apparently it can be slowed by a strong defense. One may say that increases in the rate of disease progression are more virus- dependent, while decreases are more host-dependent.

Whether sex is homosexual or heterosexual, the probability of acquiring HIV-1 is related less to promiscuity than to the type of contact and the sex of the partner. Especially among men who have sex with men, the number of partners is far less important than the kind of sex they practice. The most dangerous sex is anogenital: anal penetration by the penis. The more often an uninfected man is anally penetrated by a man infected with HIV-1, the greater his chance of acquiring HIV and AIDS, whether his partners are few or many. The safest sex is that between two women, even if they engage in anal stimulation. In fact, two women engaged in such contact (i.e., nonpenile but involving some kind of penetration) are at less risk than two men engaged in the same type of contact, possibly because force is less often a factor. HIV virulence, or damage, is directly related to its rate of circulation. This is because the virus load needed for efficient HIV transmission depends on virus reproduction within host cells that are crucial to host well-being.

The faster and more often HIV changes hosts, the more deadly it becomes. Our own studies have shown that the virus is more aggressive in times of rapid spread and less aggressive when spread is relatively slow. Spread depends on two factors: the opportunity to transmit HIV and the infectivity of the virus. Opportunity depends on the frequency of the transmission event, whether it is unprotected sex, blood transfusion, or IV drug use. Infectivity depends on the level or amount of virus in the transmitting fluid as well as the susceptibility of the host cells to that particular virus. Looking at sexual transmission (by far the most common of the three routes), we have seen that virtually all newly infected individuals have high virus loads during the first few months.

As measured by the HIV RNA in their blood, they have about equal amounts of circulating virions, making them equally HIV-infectious. But soon a distinction develops between progressors and nonprogressors (*i.e.*, those rapidly progressing to AIDS and those progressing slowly or not at all). The progressors are highly infectious due to persistent high virus loads in all their body fluids. They transmit a highly aggressive virus that reproduces fast and sustains high levels in its next host.

However, progressors are highly infectious for a relatively short time due to rapid disease progression. As their CD_4^+ cells fall, their sexual activity tends to decline because they feel increasingly ill and develop unattractive symptoms: the dark red Kaposi lesions, the continual cough of *P. carinii* pneumonia, or devastating diarrhea. In contrast, the nonprogressors are less infectious for a relatively long time because the virus load declines in their fluids. As their immune systems keep AIDS at bay, they feel healthy enough to continue sexual activity, but 'they transmit a weaker virus. It reproduces relatively slowly and cannot sustain high levels in the next host. Of course, as the epidemic continues, the progressors with their aggressive HIV contribute less and less to the viral mix. They drop out of sexual activity and ultimately die.

Therefore, we see that a new AIDS epidemic is dominated by the more infectious virus of progressors, but a late-stage epidemic is dominated by the weaker virus of nonprogressors. At times of high spread, the stronger virus shrinks the average symptom-free period because it needs less time to break down the immune system. At times of low spread, the weaker virus leads to a longer average symptom-free period. We have compelling evidence that breakdown occurs faster when HIV is acquired (by any route) from an AIDS patient whose symptom-free period was relatively short. These observations are based on various studies.

Although many gay men have stable long-term relationships, this highly active subgroup combines youthful potency with militant expression of emancipated homosexuality. Such promiscuity, practiced routinely throughout a good-sized community, may be unprecedented in history. It may be approximated by heterosexual men who continually visit many different prostitutes, but such men are rare, as far as we can tell.

For one thing, prostitutes cost money. In contrast, gay encounters in bathrooms and bathhouses are largely free of charge. Fortunately, preventive measures can reduce HIV infections and actually reverse the spiral of aggressive infection. Fewer people get HIV and AIDS. They stay healthier longer because the virus is weaker and gives them a longer symptom-free period. However, HIV remains. To keep HIV in check, everyone who is sexually active-gay or straight-must avoid the high-risk behaviour that gives HIV the advantage.

In North America and Europe, AIDS is epidemic but seems to be holding, and HIV-1 incidence has dropped. In South America and Asia, the disease is fast reaching epidemic proportions. It could easily become endemic because of factors such as poor education, communication, and medical care, which have already made it near endemic in much of Africa.

Evidence suggests that the HIV family could kill faster. It could shorten the symptom-free period that follows the initial acute infection. If so, instead of developing AIDS over several years, people might develop the disease in a matter of months. We would then see many millions more cases of AIDS than are projected on the basis of today's average disease-free period.

Outside Europe and North America, AIDS spreads mainly by heterosexual relations, perinatal infection, and conta-minated blood and hospital supplies. Control strategies must aim to safeguard the blood supplies and hospital equipment. But if HIV thrives on rapidity of consecutive transmission, these strategies will not be enough. Somehow people in Africa, Asia, and South America must be educated to lower their number of sexual partners and, even more important, their high-risk sex acts. Gay men in Amsterdam and other areas have shown this can be done.

Even in North America and Europe, HIV incidence is dropping. The decreased incidence may lead to decreased virulence and even to a weakened or attenuated virus. But virulence could just as well be boosted by ominous changes in the Western epidemic.

At first HIV-1 was spread mainly by homosexual relations, then by needle sharing among drug users. Now it is infecting more women and children, most of whom have no direct connection with drugs or homosexuals. Nature and science will hopefully ultimately show us the way, but two promising avenues have so far been disappointing.

The first involves searching the HIV family for types that are relatively harmless, either because of inherently low infectivity or loss of infectivity (attenuation). Such relatively weak viruses could give insight into more harmful types. They might ever protect us against them, as cowpox was used by Jenner to protect against smallpox. At this point, we have discovered and studied two possibilities that will later be discussed in depth.

The first is HIV type 2 (HIV-2), which emerged in the West African interior. This virus causes AIDS, but very slowly and with lower frequency than HIV-1. HIV-2 is mainly confined to West Africa, where HIV-1 subtypes are appearing with increasing frequency.

More time and study are needed to tell how well HIV-2 infection protects people against HIV-1. Although most West African AIDS victims harbor only one of the two viruses, a rare few harbor both. This could mean HIV-2 offers incomplete or temporary protection.

However, with a double infection we cannot yet tell whether the two viruses entered simultaneously or, if sequentially, which came first. We can still hope that HIV-2 has some protective potential, and new data point tentatively in that direction.

Meanwhile, HIV-1 is overtaking the slower HIV-2 in West Africa, but HIV-2 is not likely to disappear. It has a proven monkey reservoir or home base: the sooty mangabey. This monkey comfortably hosts an SIV that becomes HIV-2 when transmitted to the human body.

The new type to be studied is HIV type 0 (HIV-0). It was discovered in 1990 by Belgian researchers

Guido van der Groen and Peter Piot. Some have called it "O" for "outgroup", but "zero" is now preferred. Originally found only in Cameroon and Gabon, HIV-0 was isolated from several AIDS patients by different researchers, leaving no doubt that it can cause the disease in humans. Its virulence is unknown, but its spread is extremely limited.

The virus has just recently been seen in Europe, mainly France, in a handful of immigrants from Cameroon and Gabon. In Africa, it is only rarely seen outside its accustomed area. Even there, HIV-0 occurs in much less than 10 per cent of AIDS victims. The rest are infected with the more common HIV-1 subtypes. As with HIV-2, the closest relative to HIV-0 is not another human AIDS virus but a monkey virus. Found in chimpanzee, it is called *chimpanzee immunodeficiency virus* (CIV) or, more often, SIV cpz. Like other SIVs, it does not harm its natural host.

While HIV-2 and HIV-0 have great research value, they are not too promising as barriers against HIV-1. Though they spread and act slowly, they still cause AIDS. The second avenue is to find a virus outside the HIV family: something similar but harmless to its natural host. We have already found CIV, other SIVs and even analogs beyond the primate family. These viruses offer tantalizing clues to the HIV family. But so far, none offers us protection from HIV.

Although closely related to the killer, these viruses are remarkable and they never cause the slightest harm to their natural hosts. SIVs can even move among various types of African monkeys without harm. In fact, they seem to inhabit a different virus world than our HIV.

Without knowing the terrible AIDS story, we would never believe that these innocent monkey viruses could kill. Yet they kill humans, and some of them kill Asian monkeys. What makes these simian viruses perfectly harmless to some primates and deadly to others? How can they be so well adapted to multiply in human immune cells?

Since we find no harmless HIVs, it appears that SIV just naturally develops into an AIDS-causing pathogen after roaming from human to human for a number of viral generations. The uncertainties of human immunodeficiency virus (HIV) infection and its relentless progression to acquired immunodeficiency syndrome place enormous burden on those affected.

HIV infection drains intrapersonnel, interpersonnel and material resources and cannot be thought of as a single, stressful life event but rather as an unremitting force with uncertain course. Counsellors and therapists are not expected to be experts in the medical aspects of AIDS, it is critical that professionals who provides services to HIV-infected persons have a basic understanding of the syndrome and its manifestations. With HIV/AIDS, the emotional trauma is compounded by a societal reaction that judges the HIV-infected person very harshly, unlike current public reactions to those with heart disease or cancer. Often that severe reaction is internalized, creating a loathing of self. Consider these issues:

— Because the human immunodeficiency virus is spread through exchange of bodily fluids—during sex, in artificial insemination, when sharing contaminated syringes during injection drug use, in transfusions and infusions of blood and blood products, and from mother to baby *in utero* and during breast-feeding—HIV and AIDS is a taboo topic for many.

— Because HIV is most often spread during sex and drug use, large portions of world society judgmentally regard persons with HIV/AIDS as moral degenerates who are to blame for their illness. The judgment is evident in the allowance made for infected children and for persons who were infected by contaminated blood products, who are viewed as "innocent" victims.

— Irrational fears of contamination have deprived many of adequate medical and other care, and even from basic human contact.

Many people still believe that their communities, their family members, and they themselves are immune to HIV. But now, and especially for the next century, no individual and no community can afford to dismiss HIV as a condition that happens to others.

HIV threatens all our communities, in ways overt and in ways subtle, hidden, and complex. Mental health practitioners, especially, cannot be so dismissive or unaware. If a mental health practitioner believes HIV infection doesn't occur in his or her community and therefore fails to learn how to address it appropriately with clients, he or she does clients a grave disservice.

In fact, many would argue that discussion of HIV issues should be a part of every mental health practice. The practitioner must be able to respond empathically and skillfully to:

— Whether a person is infected with HIV or is a family member or neighbour of someone with HIV/AIDS

— When a person says a fear of HIV is preventing a desired relationship

— When a person is sexually active and doesn't fear HIV sufficiently to have safer sexual attitudes

The HIV-related tasks for mental health practitioners, then, are many and complicated. They involve constant self-scrutiny of our feelings and reactions.

They also involve constant learning. Understanding HIV entails much more than assembling a headful of facts, be they medical or psychological, to be pronounced to oneself or to a person. Skillful practice requires, foremost, a conceptualisation of HIV in which many interlocking and complicated pieces of knowledge may come together and be unified.

This conceptualisation enables the practitioner to make a comprehensive assessment of the HIV-affected person. The assessment findings and the model then guide the practitioner in planning care that is far-reaching. Finally, the model informs interdisciplinary practice, which will be a hallmark of the next decade of care. The biopsychosocial/spiritual model acknowledges that all persons have many aspects and that these aspects all interact.

These broad, interlocking aspects have the following general definitions:

— *Biological or biomedical*—pertaining to flesh, blood and bone, organisms, and entities as viruses.

— *Psychological*—having to do with the inner life of the individual, including emotions, self-judgments, motivations for relatedness with others, and internal reasons for behaviours.

— *Social*—the person's participation or lack of participation in family, community and society (including the therapist), and the effects of family, community, and society on the person. One's culture resides in this realm, although one's reactions to the culture may be psychological.

— *Spiritual*—not necessarily an attachment to organized beliefs or religious institutions, although that certainly may be present. Spiritual aspects often include an internal belief or sense that acknowledges an "other," a reality beyond normal experience, which may be a presence or meaning that surpasses current reality.

When "health care" is mentioned, for example, most people think "medical care," an indication of our overemphasis on biomedical responses, to the exclusion or neglect of care of other aspects of ourselves.

In the biopsychosocial/spiritual model, the different realms may be separated out for purposes of distinguishing major components and for planning our assessment and interventions.

Consider application of the model to the situation of a person who, after testing, is told that she is HIV-positive. Since the recognition of AIDS and HIV, and in many institutions still, the person who receives a test result that indicates HIV infection is immediately drawn into a whitewater torrent of months of laboratory tests, visits with medical providers, prescriptions for prophylactic (preventative) medicines, and discussions about the newest medical interventions.

While the body may generally be well cared for, other aspects require attention, such as:

— The person's psychological reaction. Many patients, still unfamiliar with HIV, react with the belief they have been given a death sentence. (An un-knowledgeable mental health provider may include by joining in the client's hopelessness.) Even those who cognitively "know" that HIV/AIDS is chronic are likely to have a strong psychological response that may include despair, fear, dread, guilt, shame, or even relief that comes with knowledge.

— The reactions of those who love that person, who make love with the person, go to church with the person, or are estranged from the person.

— The spiritual reaction of the person, who may or may not have a system of beliefs or feelings about God, "higher power," or meanings of life.

Social consequences may include loss of salary and of the ability to support his family, which may also affect his emotional well-being. Being sick, the man may seek a closeness to his God, or he may curse God for his situation. And what of the effects of the illness on his family, and its response?

The interplay of all these aspects is what the HIV-infected person presents to the mental health practitioner, and what must be understood as such. The biopsychosocial/spiritual model is useful because it allows us to think through what we know intuitively.

Every aspect of HIV affects and is affected by others. It allows a sophisticated response to a client who learns that he or she is HIV-positive. The practitioner who views a client as a dynamic interaction of many different aspects assumes a professional stance that responds to each component.

This response is a more comprehensive assessment that takes into account the various aspects and a treatment plan that derives from that comprehensive assessment.

In 1977 Engel used the term "biopsychosocial" and listed arguments for its adoption in medicine and psychiatry. A year later Engel alluded to an integrated model of care. He noted that the posture that science and humanism are in opposition "promotes rivalry, if not antagonism between and among health professionals.

But the care of the sick calls for collaboration and smooth interaction between professionals, with complementary roles to fulfill and tasks to perform".

This study details a biopsychosocial model based on general systems theory, taking into account culture, subculture, community, family, and intrapsychic factors, among other factors.

In the field of HIV, several persons make reference to the model, albeit from a medical vantage point. The multiple-aspects model is not just theoretical and a nice way to think about humankind. It is the basis of new ways of regarding health care, as well as of studies of mind-body connections.

Studies that acknowledge mind-body connections have emanated from scientific areas such as psychoneuroimmunology, behavioural medicine, and psychosocial oncology. More and more scientific data describe the mind-body connection.

A statistical analysis of the results of many studies in psychosocial oncology, for example, psychosocial interventions have positive effects on emotional adjustment, functional adjustment, and treatment and disease-related symptoms in adult cancer patients.

The HIV-affected person's situation—both before and after infection is complex, and the entire landscape needs to be seen and understood.

To respond in a sophisticated manner, the mental health practitioner needs to survey the entire landscape by way of a complete assessment.

1) *Medical informations*:

— Current T-helper cell counts and other markers of immune function such as viral load assays.

— Medical history, both HIV and non-HIV. An HIV-positive person may have other significant conditions, e.g., hypertension, diabetes, history of headaches.

— Medications being taken and those prescribed or recommended but declined.

— Include drugs obtained on the street, herbal remedies by nonmedical practitioners, and other comple-mentary remedies.

— Other treatments, including chiropractic care, acupuncture spiritually based healing practices.

— Self-care practices, including nutrition and exercise.

— Names of all caregivers, medical and nonmedical, include dentist, ophthalmologist, occupational therapist, physical therapist, visiting nurse, nutritionist etc. Understand their roles and the person's choices.

— Understanding of HIV-related conditions and his or h own condition.

2) *Neurological condition*

Because HIV, like certain medications, has a neurotoxic effect that affects the person's quality of life, please consider:

— Person's baseline cognitive functioning.

— Symptoms of central nervous system involvement, such as cognitive slowing, memory loss.

— Person's use of compensatory strategies, such as note taking or a reminder system.

— Peripheral nervous system involvement, indicated by pain, numbness or other symptoms in arms, hands, legs, or feet.

3) Psychological issues

- How has client's pre-HIV psychological functioning changed with knowledge of infection and progression of illness?
- Person's emotional response to HIV issues.
- Acute psychological symptoms that the client attributes to HIV status or to other stressors, *e.g.*, anxiety, unhappiness, depression, despair.
- Longstanding psychological presentation. Neglect of personality disorders severely undermines any mental health intervention and can lead practitioners to feelings of inadequacy. The personality disorders of persons must be taken into account.
- History of, and attitudes regarding, current or past experiences with mental health professionals, who may include substance abuse program counsellors; past or current participation in twelve-step programs, such as Narcotics Anonymous, Positives Anonymous.
- Use of psychiatric medications and psychoactive substances, either prescribed or obtained from street dealers. Do not overlook abuse of prescriptions and the possibilities of substance abuse in persons who do not meet your stereotype of drug abusers.
- Assess history and current sexual functioning.
- Does the client practice safer sex?
- Type of sex preferred—anal, oral, receptive?
- What has changed since diagnosis or appearance of symptoms?
- Unwanted sexual occurrences?

— If gay, lesbian, or bisexual, the person's comfort with his or her sexual preference.

4) Social issues

— For sophisticated and deeper understanding of the HIV-affected individual, strive to understand his or her culture. The person's cultural affiliations may be multiple. How does the person identify himself or herself culturally? Ask the person to explain his or her cultural identifications.

— Consider the individuals socioeconomic place in society; his or her vulnerability to racism, classism, heterosexism, and sexism; and the educational and economic opportunities denied or afforded this individual.

— Do not overlook one very important social aspect—the person's relationship with you, who becomes part of his or her social network. Note the person's ability to have a relationship with you, to accept your empathy, and to open up to you. The person's style of interaction with you is likely to mirror his or her style with similar figures outside the therapeutic relationship.

— Who are the caregivers? Does the client have two families—one of blood relatives and another of affiliation, such as friends and a partner? A genogram, or a visual display of the family, is always helpful.

— What has been the response of "family"? Consider long-time family patterns of care and current support. Are any family members likely to flee during a crisis?

— Are others in the support system HIV-positive?

— Whom does the person's designate to make treatment decisions if 'incapacitation occurs? Are the proper documents signed and filed with physicians and others? Whom should you contact in an emergency?

— Are children involved? What is their biopsychosocial status?

— What does the person want you to do if he or she misses an appointment and has no telephone or doesn't answer?

5) Spiritual issues

— History of religious observance and current attitudes.

— Person's definition, explanation, and practice of spirituality.

— Are these beliefs comforting or a source of discomfort? Do the beliefs facilitate patient's dealing with his or her HIV status or hinder it?

— With whom does the person discuss spirituality?

— What are the person's spiritual concerns?

The information gathered should be expanded to encompass the client's specific circumstances. On the basis of the information obtained through this process and your knowledge of HIV/AIDS, enter into a realistic therapeutic contract that anticipates, as well as reacts to, biopsychosocial and spiritual issues.

The mental health practitioner who uses the biopsychosocial/spiritual model acknowledges and responds to a person's many aspects. Many years of experience providing mental health services to HIV-affected persons have convinced providers that rigid frames of practice do not adequately serve clients.

The inadequacy has several causes, including these:

— Much current practice is based on Western European models, that is, white majority-culture models, of providing psychotherapy. These models are foreign to and perhaps inappropriate for minority-culture person and fail to meet their needs.

— Current psychotherapeutic models fail to account for the diverse and complex needs of medically involved patients.

While much is said about culturally sensitive or culturally competent practice, in fact it is so complicated that mental health practitioners largely ignore its implementation. Practitioners must realize that acceptance of, or sensitivity to, a person's culture is insufficient; they need to be well versed in the culture, to understand it, and to accept its role in the person's life.

The therapist must create a therapeutic relationship and make interventions that are culturally consonant for the person. Obviously, cultural competence requires a great deal of study and experience. The model provides a metamodel under which many disciplines can interact. The teamwork arises from what many of us call integrated care comes: when people talk with each other and regard each other with respect.

But, often, teamwork is hindered by a lack of a common way of thinking. Physicians, nurses, psychologists, and social workers generally emerge from training with different worldviews, including etiological presumptions, treatment strategies, and decision-making styles. The biopsychosocial/spiritual model does not require practitioners to change their worldviews. Rather, it facilitates a consensual treatment plan based on a common understanding that a person has biomedical, psychological, social, and spiritual aspects.

On the basis of that common acceptance of the model, practitioners of diverse views can sit together, view the patient in many different ways, and blend their different views into a biopsychosocial/spiritual treatment plan.

The biopsychosocial/spiritual model assists us in incorporating knowledge from other disciplines. The blending of knowledge within a system has to occur within each practitioner. What occurs when the person tells his social worker that his T-helper cell count has dropped below 200? Will the worker understand the implications and respond appropriately? Similarly, if the patient tells his physician that he takes pleasure in nothing, will the practitioner recognize a symptom of depression? Too often, we become prisoners of our training. But with the many aspects of HIV, this limitation is now insufficient for practice. To respond fully to the HIV-affected person, providers have to learn some of other disciplines' knowledge. The psychologist will never have the training of a physician, a social worker, or a member of the clergy. But he or she must be able to understand the HIV-affected person's concerns, no matter the aspect from which they come. Having a sense of other providers' knowledge allows the psychologist to work better with colleagues and extends his or her professional reach.

Barriers to the implementation of a biopsychosocial/spiritual model include the following:

— Being entrapped in one own's discipline and unwilling to extend one's breadth of knowledge.

— Adaptation of a simplistic, cartoonish view of what is meant by biopsychosocial/spiritual factors.

— Current reimbursement systems for health care, both medical and mental health. These now pressure providers to be more productive, that is, to see more patient, and therefore allow less time for inter-disciplinary meetings and discussions.

— Scepticism among patients. People who seek assistance in medical facilities generally believe that assistance comes in the form of medication. This belief requires mental health professionals in multidisciplinary programs to persuade patients of the worth of psychosocial, nonmedical services.

Biopsychosocial/spiritual model has been presented as a guide not only to understanding the condition but to assisting health care providers in structuring assessment and guiding intervention. The metamodel also informs multidisciplinary practice and encourages providers of HIV-related services to extend their knowledge beyond their disciplines. Psychiatry plays a significant role in the treatment of the immense and complex mental health needs related to HIV/AIDS. As HIV disease develops into a chronic illness, psychiatry has the opportunity to span the gulf between biological and psychosocial/spiritual approaches.

Because the virus is prevalent in groups with multiple problems, such as homelessness, chronic mental illness, and substance use, diagnosis and treatment planning become increasingly complicated. One must identify symptoms as psychiatric or neurological; although accuracy in identifying symptoms improves with time and training, diagnoses are still missed and the patient is blamed for misbehaviour. At the beginning of the HIV/AIDS epidemic, patients typically died quickly from acute infections, such as pneumocystis carinii pneumonia (PCP).

The role of psychiatrists and other mental health providers was limited, if it existed at all. As more individuals became affected, experts in the field distinguished two groups of people with HIV/AIDS and mental illness: those with pre-existing chronic and/or recurrent psychiatric illness who subsequently become HIV infected and HIV-infected persons who later develop neuropsychiatric or psychosocial problems related to their infection. Studies addressing the number of acutely hospitalized psychiatric inpatients infected with HIV-I found that between five per cent and seven per cent of individuals studied were HIV-seropositive.

Among longer-stay patients at a state hospital, HIV seroprevalence has been reported as 4 percent. Injection drug use is a well-documented risk factor for HIV infection. Several investigators have identified higher-risk behaviours among persons with mental illness, including engaging in casual sex, trading sex for money or a place to stay, combining sex with substance use, having unprotected heterosexual intercourse with known HIV-positive partners, having unprotected anal intercourse with men, and sharing needles or drug paraphernalia. The understanding of AIDS risk behaviours appears to be compromised among psychiatric inpatients. But few programs developed to date address the special needs that chronic mentally ill patients have regarding AIDS education.

In addition to prevention/education challenges, persons with mental illness who subsequently become HIV-infected also present providers with unique challenges around treatment compliance and diagnosis. What is the most effective method for keeping a homeless individual with schizophrenia and tuberculosis engaged for the several weeks to months of medications required both to ensure proper treatment of the lung infection and to minimize the risk of exposure to the general population? Are the current psychiatric symptoms seen in an immunocompromised patient an exacerbation of bipolar disorder or indicative of a central nervous system infection? The World Health Organization Neuropsychiatric AIDS Study, which attempted to study a population representative of the current epidemic, reported a higher prevalence of current mental disorders among symptomatic HIV-1 infected persons than among HIV-1 seronegative controls. AIDS dementia, characterized by cognitive impairment, motor dysfunction, and changes in mood/personality, typically occurs in significantly immunocompromised AIDS patients. Earlier reports suggested a prevalence at a single point in time from 8 per cent to 16 percent, with prevalence over the life of the individual approaching 40 to 50 percent. More recent studies suggest that this illness occurs in 10 to 20 per cent of AIDS patients.

Delirium, defined as an acute confusional state with a physiological cause, is characterized by disturbances of consciousness and attention, changes in cognition or perceptual disturbances, and acute onset with a fluctuating course. Many providers mistake delirium for dementia. Many take it for granted as a natural part of dying. Misconceptions result in underrecognition and inappropriate treatment of this condition. In one study of hospitalized AIDS patients, delirium accounted for 57 per cent of the identifiable organic mental disorders seen in the study group.

The study also includes reports of other neurological diseases presenting with psychiatric symptoms: toxoplasmosis and psychosis; cryptococcal meningitis and mania; dementia and depression.

Adequate population-based descriptive studies that outline the frequency and the severity of psychiatric illness in HIV/AIDS patients, and the subsequent effect of such an illness on function and general health, remain missing from the literature. In addition to neuropsychiatric illness, mental health providers working with HIV/AIDS patients commonly address spiritual or existential crises across the spectrum of HIV disease.

Farmer and Kleinman describe AIDS as human suffering despite the rational-technical language of disease. Kuhn advocates viewing spirituality as a legitimate and purposeful area of medical investigation. Psychiatrists working in the area of HIV/AIDS certainly possess a unique role in overseeing psychopharma-cological interventions. Unfortunately, much of the literature in this area consists of anecdotal information and case reports.

Only recently have controlled medication trials in HIV/ AIDS patients for common psychiatric illnesses such as depression been published. The unique role of psychiatry in the treatment of HIV/AIDS patients encompasses and balances each aspect of the biopsychosocial/spiritual model; the psychiatrist is at once physician, consultant/liaison, educator, therapist, and visionary.

3

Sexually Transmitted Diseases (STDs)

Sexually transmitted diseases (STDs) are passed from one person to another by sexual contact. Specifically, an STD may be passed on to someone if they are exposed to infected body fluids (such as semen or vaginal fluid, and sometimes blood) during vaginal intercourse, anal intercourse and sometimes during oral sex. STDs have traditionally been regarded as unmentionable and something to be ashamed of because of the generally negative attitude to sexual matters found in most societies. There has often been an assumption that infection with an STD implies that a person is promiscuous and deserves to get an infection because of their immoral behaviour.

This sort of attitude has been seen recently in descriptions of AIDS as a 'gay plague', as if it were a punishment for homosexual behaviour. The reality is, however, that STDs are diseases like any others. They simply happen to be passed on by sexual activity. Some STDs are more infectious than others, although anyone—regardless of sex, class, age, ethnic background or wealth —may develop an STD if he or she has sexual contact with a sexual partner and is not protected by the use of a condom.

An STD requires medical treatment. Left untreated, STDs may cause further complications. Unfortunately, some STDs can be present, especially in women, without causing symptoms. This is why it is important for people with STD symptoms to let their partners know, so that they can get treatment as well. If a man or woman thinks they may have an STD, they should visit a GUM (genito-urinary medicine) clinic (formerly known as STD or special clinics). These are normally found at hospitals.

Trained staff will make a diagnosis—it may not be an STD—and prescribe a course of treatment that should clear up the infection. They will also help the patient psychologically and enable their partner (contact) or partners to be traced if necessary, tested and treated. This is all done in a confidential and discreet manner. To reduce the risk of contracting STDs —apart from complete abstinence—it is advisable always to practise safer sex by using a condom.

This applies as much to long-term relationships as it does to casual sex. People do get STDs in long-term relationships even when both partners are claiming that they are monogamous. Considered first in this section is HIV, a virus which can be transmitted sexually, and which eventually causes AIDS.

HIV and AIDS

HIV (human immunodeficiency virus) is a virus that attacks the immune system and can eventually cause AIDS (acquired immune deficiency syndrome), a syndrome that was first identified in 1981. HIV, recognized as the causative agent in 1983, is commonly passed on by sexual intercourse through body fluids such as blood, semen and vaginal secretions. In addition, HIV can be passed on by injecting equipment (needles and unsterilized syringes) shared by drug users, infected blood in transfusions, from infected mothers to newborn babies and (less commonly) by blood contact through open cuts.

At present HIV appears to be incurable and, over time, causes the body's natural defence system to stop functioning so that the carrier becomes prey to one or more opportunistic diseases which eventually cause death (although new therapies are allowing people with HIV to live much longer). If a person has HIV and one or more of these diseases, they are diagnosed as having AIDS.

The most encouraging aspect is that people can considerably reduce the risk of contracting HIV and developing AIDS by altering their sexual behaviour and practising 'safer sex'. It has to be remembered, however, that once a person has HIV, he or she may pass it on to another person at any time if they have unsafe sex. AIDS in Europe and North America appeared to be confined mainly to homosexual and bisexual men and intravenous drug users.

But the number of men and women who have contracted HIV through heterosexual sex has increased in Europe and North America, and AIDS has become a major cause of death among young people in their twenties and thirties. In Africa, however, HIV has from the very start spread mainly through the heterosexual population, probably because the predominant HIV sub-type in this part of the world is 'better' at infecting the cells that line the vagina.

By the end of 1994, the WHO (World Health Organization) estimated that worldwide approximately 4.5 million people had developed AIDS. With no cure in sight at present, it has become clear that people need to be aware that they are at risk of developing an HIV infection if they have unprotected sex. This is a point that parents and teachers could raise with children when they talk to them about HIV and AIDS, and about sexually transmitted diseases in general. AIDS is caused by the human immunodeficiency virus (HIV), which can be transmitted in body fluids—primarily blood, semen and vaginal secretions —that enter the body during sexual contact, through small cuts or lesions in the skin, or via the tissue lining the internal parts of the reproductive system.

The chances of contracting HIV through unprotected anal intercourse— where delicate tissues are more likely to tear—are much higher than through vaginal intercourse. The risk is also greater if other STDs that cause breaks in the skin, such as herpes, are already present.

To understand how HIV infects the body, and how AIDS develops, it helps to understand, in simple terms, the workings of the body's immune system. Throughout its life, the human body faces an onslaught of disease-causing microorganisms, including bacteria and viruses, attempting to enter the body.

Those that penetrate the first line of defences—such as the skin—are then detected and destroyed by the immune system. This system consists of billions of cells that enable us to fight off infections. Some, called macro-phages, roam through the bloodstream and tissues in search of invading microorganisms and eat them.

Macrophages also 'Inform' other cells of the immune system that there are invaders inside the body. First on the scene are the helper T-cells which alert the entire immune system to launch an all-out attack on the specific invader. This includes the production of 'killer chemicals' called antibodies that help to wipe out microorganisms. This is what normally happens when infections threaten, but when HIV invades the body things seem to go wrong.

All viruses need to enter living cells in order to reproduce. The cells that HIV selects for invasion are the helper T-cells, key elements in the immune response. HIV viruses take over the genetic material of these cells and replicate themselves, destroying the helper T-cells in the process. Although the body produces antibodies to combat the growing HIV menace, the immune system is gradually worn down over the years as the number of key helper T-cells decreases. This is the stage at which AIDS develops.

Lacking its normal defences, the body is vulnerable to infection by opportunistic diseases that would normally be repelled by a healthy immune system. Eventually, one or more of these diseases completely overwhelms the body, leading to the death of the AIDS sufferer.

There is no conclusive proof that all people infected with HIV will necessarily go on to develop AIDS. Since the disease was only identified relatively recently, long-term studies have not yet been able to identify which of the people who are HIV-positive will not develop AIDS. However, men and women who are infected with HIV, and who do develop AIDS, typically progress through four noticeable stages.

— Stage 1—*Initial acute infection*: Up to a quarter of people show initial symptoms between two and five weeks after infection with HIV. These symptoms can include general body aches, sore throat, fever, chills, widespread rash, oral and genital ulceration and swollen lymph glands. However, it is very important to realize that these are non-specific symptoms which could indicate other mild viral infections apart from HIV.

— *Stage 2—Asymptomatic HIV infection*: During the asymptomatic (without symptoms) phase, which lasts on average up to 10 years or longer, a person looks and feels completely healthy, although the virus is actively replicating inside the body. But he or she may suffer from lymphadenopathy: swelling of the lymph nodes (or glands)—centres for fighting infections—found in the neck, armpits and groin.

During this phase a person is infective and may pass on the virus to other people without realizing that he or she is infected. Why this phase varies in length between different individuals is not yet clear, although it probably depends on a number of factors, including age, lifestyle and the presence of other infections. Some people— known as non-progressors—have remained symptom-free for many years, and only time will tell if they will ever develop AIDS. If they do not, it may be the result of their particular lifestyle, the type of HIV they were infected with, or the potency of their individual immune system.

— *Stage 3 - Symptomatic HIV infection:* The onset of this symptomatic phase indicates that the immune system is weakening under the HIV onslaught, making the body more susceptible to diseases which would normally be controlled. These include the fungal infection thrush (candidiasis) in the mouth— in healthy women thrush is a common infection of the vagina. Other common symptoms are skin complaints, weight loss, bouts of tiredness, diarrhoea and sweating.

— *Stage 4—Advanced symptoms*: AIDS As the immune system weakens further, the symptoms of AIDS develop. There is a fixed set of symptoms and diseases that characterize the syndrome. Some are worsening of the symptoms experienced during symptomatic HIV infection: fevers and night sweats, and progressive weight loss. Opportunistic infections, such as *Pneumocystis carinii pneumonia* (PCP), extensive herpes, tuberculosis or encephalitis, which eventually prove fatal, are also AIDS-defining. HIV may infect brain c too, causing dementia. Once a person has AIDS—with one or more of these specific conditions and HIV—it will probably prove fatal at some time in the next four years.

If someone is worried that they may have been infected with HIV, there are a number of people to talk to. There is no point in waiting and worrying needlessly. A helpline such as that run by the Terrence Higgins Trust or the National Aids Helpline might be the first stop. At a GUM clinic or at an HIV/AIDS advice centre, there should be a counsellor or doctor with whom to talk through the issues, to discuss the possible advantages and disadvantages of testing, and to enable someone to come to an informed decision as to whether or not to take a test to see if they have an HIV infection.

It may help to talk to a friend or relative, if they are sympathetic and can be trusted to keep a confidence. If a person does decide to be tested, a blood sample is taken and sent to a laboratory for testing. The blood test identifies the presence or absence of antibodies against HIV If the test is negative it means that the person is probably not infected with HIV, although antibodies can take some time to appear in the blood (more than six weeks) and a further, later blood test may be suggested.

If the test is positive, it will be repeated with a more sensitive test to check its correctness before the patient is informed of the result. If it is still positive it means that the person is infected with HIV—they are HIV-positive. Once the test result comes through, a doctor or counsellor at the clinic will inform a patient in person whether the test was positive or negative. Not surprisingly, many people react with shock and despair when they discover they are HIV-positive. Usually clinic staff will refer them to suitable counsellors and self-help groups. If an individual has told his or her trustworthy friends or relatives, they can be of great help in providing support, and helping to plan for the future, although unfortunately some people have a more hostile reaction.

At the time of writing there is no cure for HIV infection or AIDS, although treatments have been used to alleviate the effects of both. Since the late 1980s, the drug AZT has been used to slow the progression of HIV infection, although recent research has shown that its benefits may be limited when used alone. However, many centres use AZT as part of a cocktail of drugs (combination therapy) employed to inhibit the development of the HIV infection. Patients also receive antibiotics to prevent AIDS-related infections. People with symptomatic HIV or with full-blown AIDS are given specific treatment according to the condition, although there comes a time when the infections are no longer treatable.

Chlamydia

This is the general name for infections caused by the bacteria-like organism *Chlamydia trachomatis*. Chlamydial infections occur in both men and women and are transmitted mainly by vaginal intercourse, or less commonly by anal intercourse or oral sex. *C. trachomatis is* the main infective agent in mucopurulent cervicitis (MPC) in women and non-gonococcal urethritis (NGU) in men. A high proportion of women with chlamydia do not have MPC or any of its symptoms.

— *Mucopurulent cervicitis (MPC):* This inflammation of the cervix is most often caused by *Chlamydia trachomatis*, but it can also be caused by *Neisseria gonorrhoeae* (the bacterium that causes gonorrhoea). The main symptom of MPC is a discharge from the cervix, although many women do not notice that it is any different from a normal vaginal discharge. If MPC is diagnosed (by seeing a red cervix and pus discharge), it can be treated with antibiotics. Untreated, C. *trachomatis* and other microorganisms that cause MPC can spread to other parts of the reproductive system and may cause pelvic inflammatory disease.

— *Non-gonococcal urethritis (NGU)*: NGU, one of the commonest male STDs, is an inflammation of the male urethra produced by microorganisms other than the bacterium that causes gonorrhoea. Over 50 percent of cases of NGU are caused by *Chlamydia trachomatis*. Symptoms of NGU include a clear or pus-like discharge from the penis; and pain or a burning feeling when urinating. Some men, however, have very mild symptoms or none at all. NGU is usually treated by antibiotics, although the type of treatment depends on what type of agent has caused the disease. Female partners should also be treated, as transmission of NGU may cause MPC or PID, and the couple should refrain from sexual contact until both of them are cured. Untreated, NGU can cause painful inflammation of the epididymis (part of the testis) or a urethral stricture, a narrowing of the urethra.

Genital herpes

This sexually transmitted disease produces sporadic outbreaks of painful blisters on the genitals. It is caused mainly by the herpes simplex type two virus. Once a person has become infected by herpes simplex, the virus stays inside the body for life, although it may remain inactive for much or all of that time, and some infected people never show any symptoms at all. Genital herpes is highly infectious. Usually a person contracts the disease through sexual contact with a partner who has the blisters on their genitals.

However, it appears that the virus may sometimes be passed on by someone who is infected but shows no outwards signs of infection. Oral sex may sometimes cause infection if the person performing the act has cold sores, as may use of infected sex toys, such as vibrators. Some three to six days after infection, a person who develops symptoms of herpes first feels irritation or burning in the genitals before small, clear blisters appear on the penis or vulva. These blisters burst open to leave painful ulcers which will heal within 10-21 days. This first episode of herpes is often accompanied by high temperature, headaches and muscle pains. Sufferers may experience a burning feeling during urination and women may have a discharge. After this first occurrence of herpes, one-third of sufferers have no further flare-ups, another third have a few further episodes, and the remaining third have frequent attacks—more than three times a year.

Recurrences may be triggered by sunbathing, stress or sometimes sexual intercourse. A tingling feeling in the genitals is often an early warning sign that an attack is about to start. Subsequent attacks may be less painful than the first because the body starts to build up resistance, but men and women who experience repeated occurrences of genital herpes commonly find the condition distressing and painful. There is no 'cure' for genital herpes because the virus cannot be eliminated. If a sexual partner has been diagnosed as having genital herpes, condoms should always be used to prevent infection of the other partner. However, the antiviral drug acyclovir is very effective in reducing the pain and duration of the first attack. In patients with frequent, long-term attacks, the use of acyclovir will reduce or abolish the attacks while the drug is taken.

Genital herpes passed from a mother to her newborn child can cause severe illness and possibly death. For this reason, mothers who suffer an attack when they are about to give birth may be delivered by caesarean section and acyclovir given to the infant. Along with antiviral drugs, there are several self-help strategies that may help alleviate the effects of an attack of genital herpes. Avoid sexual contact during an attack and until two or three days after blisters have healed completely.

— Wear loose-fitting cotton underwear.

— Take aspirin or ibuprofen to reduce pain.

— Wash the genitals regularly during an infection and pat them dry with a towel—this should be washed afterwards.

— Wash hands carefully after touching the affected area, in order to avoid spreading the infection to other parts of the body.

— After swimming, do not sit around wearing damp swimwear.

Genital warts

Genital warts appear on the genitals or around the anus and must be treated medically. Soft and generally painless, genital warts range in form from individual small, flat bumps to pink or greyish-white growths that resemble tiny cauliflowers and can form an extensive covering.

Genital warts are caused by certain types of the human papilloma virus (HPV) that can be transmitted by sexual contact. Over 60 percent of partners of individuals who have genital warts will develop the disease. However, it may take weeks, months or even years before signs and symptoms appear, and even before they do, the virus can be passed on to a new partner. Sufferers may experience embarrassment about their warts, and possibly discomfort. They should, however, seek treatment as soon as possible.

In addition, women should seek diagnosis if their partner has genital warts because, even if they themselves show no signs of infection, the warts may be concealed inside the vagina or on the cervix. Various types of treatment are available, including application of poclophyllin, a caustic chemical which erodes the warts (not to be used for pregnant women); liquid nitrogen, which is used to freeze the warts; or laser treatment to burn away the warts.

However, no treatment can remove the virus from the body; it remains inactive within body tissues, but it may reactivate and genital warts may recur. As well as seeking treatment, a woman who has had genital warts—or whose partner has had them—should also have regular cervical smear tests because there is evidence that women infected with certain types of HPV have an increased risk of developing cervical cancer.

Gonorrhoea

Gonorrhoea is one of the commonest STDs worldwide, although it is becoming uncommon in most Western countries. It is a highly infectious disease caused by the bacterium *Neisseria gonorrhoeae*, which affects more men than women and is more prevalent among teenagers and young adults, especially those with numerous sexual partners. It is usually passed on by anal, vaginal or oral sex. Symptoms of gonorrhoea, when they occur, appear within two days to two weeks of getting the infection.

Male symptoms include a burning feeling on urination, followed by a milky discharge from the penis, which becomes thicker. However, some 10 percent of men and 50 percent of women show no initial symptoms. Untreated, gonorrhoea may spread to the prostate gland or the epididymis of the testis, causing inflammation and, possibly in the latter case, permanent sterility, although this is now rare. Women infected with gonorrhoea may also feel burning when urinating, although the most usual symptoms are vaginal discharge, dyspareunia (painful sexual intercourse) and pelvic pain. But about half of all women infected with gonorrhoea show no symptoms, or have symptoms so mild that they ignore them.

Even when symptoms are present, they are so non-specific that they could be confused with other infections such as cystitis. The problem is that, left untreated, the bacteria that cause gonorrhoea can travel through the reproductive system and cause PID, which can have serious consequences, including infertility. For this reason it is vital that, should a man discover he has gonorrhoea, he must tell his female partner or partners that they may have the infection, because it may remain hidden inside their body and cause further damage. Once diagnosed by taking a smear of discharge for microscopic examination, gonorrhoea is treated with a course of antibiotics. Women may also be given antibiotics that eliminate any chlamydia infection around a quarter of people with gonorrhoea also have chlamydia.

Hepatitis B

Hepatitis is an inflammation of the liver caused by a number of different viruses. Hepatitis B is a form of the disease caused by the hepatitis B virus (HBV). A person infected with hepatitis may show no symptoms, but if symptoms do develop they usually include a flu-like illness, fever, loss of appetite, nausea, possibly jaundice (a yellowing of the skin and eyes) and a feeling of tenderness in the upper abdomen. Usually the illness subsides after about three weeks and the liver returns to normal functioning within a few months. One of the major routes of transmission of hepatitis B is through sexual activity, including oral sex and kissing. It can also be transmitted via blood, shared needles, unsterile tattooing and earpiercing, as well as from a mother to her newborn infant via her milk.

The reason for this is that the HBV can be found in most of the bodily fluids of an infected person, including semen, saliva and vaginal secretions, and it is highly infectious. The HBV can also be passed on from mother to foetus. Hepatitis B was once more common among male homosexuals, although it appears that heterosexual intercourse is now the main route for the sexual transmission of HBV, with having many partners the main risk factor.

If a doctor suspects that a patient may have hepatitis B, he or she will confirm it by means of a blood test. There is no specific treatment for hepatitis B, although rest, a good diet and avoiding alcohol should aid recovery. Vaccination against hepatitis B is available, but at present it is targeted at those most at risk, such as doctors, nurses, people with multiple sexual partners such as prostitutes, and intravenous drug users. In 5-10 percent of cases, the HBV persists and the person becomes a carrier, able to pass on the disease but not showing any symptoms. Carriers may also risk developing other liver disease, such as cancer, which may lead to death.

Pelvic inflammatory disease (PID)

Pelvic inflammatory disease (PID) is an inflammation of the female reproductive organs, especially the ovaries, fallopian tubes and uterus, and is a common cause of lower abdominal pain in women. It is most common in younger, sexually active women, and it has a higher incidence in women who use the IUD as a contraceptive. PID is often caused by a sexually transmitted disease that has not been treated, often because it has shown no symptoms.

Women with PID may have pain in the abdominal or pelvic regions, especially during or just after sex. They may also develop a fever or backache and have irregular periods. However, many women with PID show no symptoms. Once diagnosed, PID is treated immediately with antibiotics; specific antibiotics can be prescribed once the microorganism(s) causing the infection have been identified.

Present and past sexual partners should also be treated to prevent further cases of infection. In more serious cases of PID, women are often admitted to hospital for treatment. Left untreated, PID can cause infertility, or increase the risk of ectopic pregnancy—a pregnancy occurring inside the fallopian tube which has to be terminated to avoid harming the mother.

Pubic lice

Many parents are familiar with head lice—tiny insects that bite into the scalp and feed on blood—either because their children have had them or because they themselves had them as children. Another species of these tiny insects lives on and among the pubic hair of adults, feeding on blood and causing irritation and itching.

Pubic lice are also known as crab lice or crabs because they have 'claws' which they use to grip the shafts of pubic hair in order to avoid being dislodged. Pubic lice are usually transmitted by sexual contact—they simply move from one person's pubic hair to his or her partner's—although they may also be spread by infected sheets or towels. Infection can be confirmed by inspecting the pubic hair. If the pinhead-sized lice cannot be seen, their white eggs—called nits—may be visible, attached to the pubic hairs. Normal bathing or showering will not remove lice or their eggs. A special shampoo that contains insecticide is needed to do this.

Syphilis

Once a widespread and much-feared disease, syphilis is now less common because of effective treatment, although it is still a serious illness. In recent times, localized outbreaks of the disease have occurred among some groups of drug users who have turned to prostitution on a large scale to finance their habit.

Primary and secondary syphilis are highly infectious and can be transmitted by most forms of sexual contact with an infected person including oral sex and kissing. Syphilis can also be transmitted across the placenta from mother to foetus, although this is now less common because of routine testing for syphilis during pregnancy. Syphilis is caused by the bacterium *Treponema pallidum*, which remains in the body indefinitely if not treated, causing a disease that follows three distinct stages.

The symptom of primary syphilis, which appears between 10 and 90 days after infection, is a painless ulcer that appears at the site of exposure—either on the genitals or around the anus or mouth—and heals within 6-10 weeks. In the following weeks, secondary syphilis develops. Its symptoms can include skin rashes, headache. sore throat, enlarged lymph nodes, mild fever, hair loss and flattened, wartlike growths that occur on moist areas around the genitals and anus.

These symptoms disappear within a few weeks or months, and a person moves into the latent, symptomless phase of the disease. Some years after infection, some untreated people develop the tertiary, and most destructive, stage of the disease. Its effects include damage to the brain and nervous system, and to the cardiovascular (blood) system, which may cause mental disorders or even death. Progression to the latent and tertiary phases is unusual, however. If syphilis is diagnosed—by a blood test—in its primary, secondary or latent stages, the disease can be treated effectively with the antibiotic penicillin.

Trichomoniasis

Trichomoniasis is caused by *Tricbomonas vaginalis*, which belongs to a group of microorganisms called protists. Symptoms of trichomoniasis include painful irritation of the vulva and vagina; an excessive, yellow, frothy discharge, with a foul smell; and possibly pain on urination. Some women show no symptoms, and T vaginalis may live inside the vagina for some time without causing infection and then suddenly flare up and produce trichomoniasis symptoms. Although the disease is sexually transmitted, men rarely show symptoms. So a man may unwittingly pass on the disease, picked up months or years previously, to a new female partner, and she might erroneously think he has been unfaithful. Some men, however, develop NGU as a result of infection.

Non-sexually transmitted diseases

Many people feel unnecessarily confused and ashamed if they develop a sexual infection and may be too embarrassed to consult a doctor. The description of sexual infections that follows is not intended to be a guide to self-diagnosis. If you or your sexual partner show signs or symptoms of a sexual infection or irritation, you should consult your doctor or visit a hospital genito-urinary medicine (GUM) clinic as soon as possible to obtain an accurate diagnosis.

Doctors and nurses who treat sexual diseases are used to seeing people who have—or turn out not to have—these infections. They will not be embarrassed, patronizing or judgmental. Their job is to treat a patient with a sexual infection in the same way that an orthopaedic surgeon would treat someone with a broken leg. Ignoring a sexual infection or irritation will not make it go away. Nor will it do any good to blame a partner for passing on a disease that may not even be present. It may well be the case that the infection has not been passed on sexually or that it is non-infectious.

These are sexual infections that are not generally transmitted by sexual contact and that mainly affect women (usually in the urinary tract). So what causes them? On the skin, and inside certain body openings, such as the mouth, vagina, rectum and anus, a community of microorganisms including bacteria and fungi live quite harmlessly, keeping each other in check and stopping any one type of microorganism from taking over. This is much like a cultivated garden where different types of plants co-existbut prevent any one variety from dominating. In fact, the community of bacteria and fungi on or in the body is often described as a 'flora'. But sometimes things go wrong. Bacteria that are harmless in the rectum, for example, might be accidentally transferred to the vagina, where they cause infection.

Alternatively, the vaginal flora might be disrupted so that one microorganism grows out of control and causes an infection. Non-sexually transmitted diseases can occur in women of all ages, who may or may not be sexually active. Vaginal and urinary infections cause discomfort to many women, and are among the most common gynaecological complaints that women see their doctors about.

Acute urethral syndrome

This is a condition that affects the urethra (the tube that carries urine from the bladder) in women. Common symptoms include a frequent urge to urinate, a feeling of discomfort in the lower part of the stomach, and pain around the vulva. It may be caused by infection of the urethra by bacteria from the large intestine, in which case it can be treated with antibiotics and by drinking plenty of water. Alternatively it may, in women who have gone through the menopause, be caused by an inflammation of the vulva which can be treated with hormonal creams. However, in a large proportion of women the cause is unknown.

Bacterial vaginosis

Bacterial vaginosis (BV) is an infection of the vagina that occurs in sexually active women. Its main symptoms are the presence of a greyish-white, often frothy vaginal discharge that has a fishy odour, and sometimes mild irritation and burning in the vagina and vulva.

BV is caused by a disturbance in the vaginal flora: naturally protective bacteria decrease in number, while others undergo a 'population explosion' that produces the symptoms of vaginosis. This bacterial imbalance is believed to be caused by sexual activity, but is not sexually transmitted. BV is treated by antibiotics, either taken by mouth or introduced in cream or gel form into the vagina.

Cystitis

Cystitis is an inflammation of the bladder, normally caused by bacterial infection. It is common in women of all ages and can be irritating and annoying, especially if it lasts for long periods.

The main symptoms are a frequent urge to urinate, although only releasing a small amount of urine each time; and a burning or stinging feeling during urination. This happens because the inflammation of the bladder's interior prevents the complete emptying of the bladder during urination, allowing infective bacteria to multiply in the urine stagnating in the bladder and urethra.

The bladder and urethra are normally free of any microorganisms. The bacteria that cause cystitis are unwanted invaders either from the vagina or from the rectum via the anus. They are accidentally introduced into the entrance of the urethra from the vulva, where there may be various bacteria present, and travel up to the bladder.

Cystitis is much more common in women than men because the female urethra is much shorter than the male's, so bacteria do not have far to travel to the bladder. Movement of bacteria into the urethra may be assisted by sexual intercourse. Cystitis can often disappear of its own accord. If symptoms persist beyond 48 hours, or if they are severe—especially if the urine is foul-smelling or tinged with blood, or if a woman has a chill or fever—she should consult her doctor.

If bacterial cystitis has been confirmed—by taking a urine sample—a doctor will prescribe antibiotics to remove the infective bacteria. If left untreated, the bacteria may spread to the kidneys and cause pyelonephritis, an inflammation of the kidneys, which is far more serious. Self-help remedies for cystitis include drinking plenty of water at regular intervals during the day to flush out the urinary system, and over-the-counter preparations of potassium citrate. Women who are sexually active and prone to cystitis may find it helpful to urinate before and after intercourse to flush out any bacteria.

Thrush

Thrush is an infection of the vagina. Like cystitis, it can occur in women of all ages, sexually active or not. Symptoms typically include a thick, white vaginal discharge, rather like cottage cheese, which has a yeasty smell; vaginal irritation and itching; and, possibly, a burning feeling in the vagina if a woman has sexual intercourse.

Thrush is caused by a yeast-like fungus, called *Candida albicans*, found in the vagina, vulva, rectum and mouth, and on the skin. As part of the natural vaginal flora, *C. albicans is* normally prevented from spreading excessively by vaginal bacteria. But sometimes the vaginal flora is disrupted and the fungus grows uncontrollably to produce thrush symptoms. Usually this happens because the vaginal environment is altered—for example, by taking antibiotics to control a bacterial infection which also kill vaginal bacteria; by using certain types of combined oral contraceptive pill; or by becoming pregnant. Thrush may also occur where the body's immune system is weakened by stress; by the long-term use of corticosteroid drugs; or in people suffering from AIDS or diabetes.

Occasionally, men develop thrush after intercourse with an infected partner, as indicated by inflammation of the glans of the penis. Treatment involves the use of an antifungal drug. For women, this usually takes the form of a pessary or cream to be inserted into the vagina, and possibly as a cream to be applied to the vulva.

Doctors may also prescribe a cream for a male partner to apply to his penis to prevent possible reinfection. A natural remedy that may help to treat thrush is the use of natural yoghurt containing live bacteria, *Lactobacillus acidopbilus*. Some yoghurt should be applied inside the vagina and left for at least two hours.

During infection it may be preferable to refrain from intercourse— this may be painful in any case— or to use a condom. Thrush can grow in the mouth, so oral sex should also be avoided until treatment is completed.

Vaginitis

Vaginitis is a general term which describes the uncomfortable, irritating and sometimes painful condition caused by inflammation of the vagina, which may also produce an abnormal and excessive vaginal discharge. It may be caused by thrush or by a sexually transmitted disease called trichomoniasis both conditions that require medical treatment. Alternatively, vaginitis can be a non-infectious disease, resulting from an allergy to a spermicide, irritation by soaps or bath oils, or the use of vaginal deodorants. In all these cases, alleviation of symptoms can be achieved by avoiding using particular products.

Drugs addiction and sex disorders

There are hundreds of different drugs available to us. We take some—including alcohol, cigarettes, caffeine (in coffee and tea), cannabis and other 'soft' drugs—to help us relax or to relieve stress; these all have some sort of physiological effect. We take other drugs—including tranquillizers, sleeping pills and numerous other prescribed drugs—to help relieve pain, or to cure or relieve the symptoms of an illness or disease. Unknown to many people, a number of prescription drugs may affect their sex lives (for instance, by reducing their desire for sex, reducing a woman's vaginal lubrication, or making it difficult for a man to obtain an erection) especially if the drugs are taken over a prolonged period.

If a man or woman feels that a prescribed drug may be affecting their sexuality, they should consult their doctor to find out whether there is any alternative type of medication available. All of us are aware that some drugs can damage our health in either a general or specific way. Unfortunately, there is so much ignorance and fear surrounding the question of drugs and how they can affect different individuals or groups of people that many people are unaware—or alternatively exaggerate—how a drug can affect their health.

One of the most common legal drugs in use and abuse is ethanol, better known as alcohol and found in a number of forms, including wine, beer and whisky. Physiologically, alcohol is a depressant of the central nervous system, the body's control and coordination centre.

Initially the effect is one of relaxation, but as the amount of alcohol in the blood increases, a person typically becomes more uninhibited and starts to lose motor (movement) control, until, if they get very drunk, they suffer memory loss and blackouts and may even finally fall into a coma. Drinking may make people believe that they 'feel' more sexual and are more ready to take part in sexual acts, but it makes them physiologically less sexual. In men, alcohol suppresses erections and causes retarded (late) ejaculation; when copious amounts of alcohol have been consumed, there may be—despite the desire—no erection at all.

Many women apparently feel sexier the more they drink, despite the fact that physiologically the opposite seems to be occurring: alcohol reduces blood flow to the vagina and vulva, delays orgasms, makes the orgasm less intense, and interferes with vaginal lubrication. Chronic alcohol use and alcohol addiction can cause all types of sexual problems. In men it can cause loss of erection, failure to ejaculate, and loss of libido (sex drive), possibly as a result of the testes shrinking and production of the male hormone testosterone decreasing.

Nicotine, the principal active agent in tobacco, is a highly addictive drug. Apart from significantly increasing the risk of lung cancer and fatal heart disease, cigarette smoking causes a wide range of other harmful effects on the body, including some that affect an individual's sex life.

— Heavy smokers generally smell and taste of cigarette smoke and are therefore less attractive in terms of basic hygiene.

— Women smokers have an increased risk of developing cervical cancer.

— Women smokers who are on the Pill and are overweight are more likely to develop a thrombosis.

— Women smokers who are pregnant may adversely affect the health of their developing child.

— Smoking makes skin age more rapidly.

— Men who smoke heavily may find it difficult to attain or maintain an erection.

Although many illegal drugs are often thought to have an aphrodisiac effect, the opposite is often true.

GUM clinics

Genito-urinary medicine (GUM) clinics (special clinics) provide expert advice, diagnosis and treatment for suspected sexually transmitted diseases. Typically, they do not require referral of a patient from another doctor; the patient simply turns up at the clinic. Attitudes towards STDs and their treatment have been transformed in recent years. Today, with far less stigma attached to them, a more enlightened attitude is taken towards STDs, and this is reflected in the workings of GUM clinics. The welcoming, relaxed atmosphere found in the majority of GUM clinics puts most people at their ease. Information about individual patients is always treated as totally confidential, and in some cases clinic staff refer to patients by a number rather than their name in order to preserve their anonymity.

Health advisers and psychologists are available to help patients deal with the psychological aspects of sexual infections such as the HIV virus and genital herpes. After an initial examination by a doctor who specializes in STDs, the patient is given a full set of tests to screen for a number of different STDs. This is because, even when a patient only appears to have symptoms of one particular STD, that STD may be accompanied by others even though the symptoms of any other STDs may not be clear. Testing may involve taking a sample from inside the vagina or from the cervix, or just inside the male urethra—the tube that runs inside the penis. Or it may require a urine sample or a blood test. If an STD is diagnosed, then treatment can begin. This often takes the form of antibiotics, but again, it depends on the particular disease.

4

AIDS and Breast-feeding

Mother-to-child transmission of the virus—during pregnancy, delivery or breastfeeding—is responsible for more than 90 per cent of HIV infection in children. Of those infants who are infected through MTCT, it is believed that about two-thirds are infected during pregnancy and around the time of delivery, and about one-third are infected through breast-feeding.

Breast-feeding is normally the best way to feed infants, its benefits go beyond sound nutrition, and children should not needlessly be deprived of it. Breast milk provides, in an easily digested form, all the nutrients an infant requires for at least the first four months of life, and usually for six months. From the moment of birth, breast milk actively protects infants against infection. It contains numerous anti-infective factors, including immunoglobulins and white blood cells, and growth factors which stimulate the development of the infant's gut. No artificial foods contain these anti-infective and growth factors. Some studies show that even with optimal hygiene, artificially fed infants suffer five times the rate of diarrhoeal infection of breast-fed infants, and higher rates of respiratory, ear and other infections. A study in a situation of poor hygiene found that the risk of death from diarrhoea in artificially fed infants was 14 times that of breast-fed infants.

Breast milk continues to provide high quality nutrients and helps to protect against some forms of infection until a child is at Least two years old. From 6 to 12 months, breast-feeding can provide up to half or more, and from 12 to 24 months up to one-third, of a child's nutrient requirements. Family planning: Breast-feeding delays the return of a woman's fertility. If a woman does not breast-feed, she is at increased risk of an early pregnancy. It is important to ensure that she has access to appropriate contraceptives within six weeks of delivery.

Breast-feeding is important to the emotional relationship, or bonding, between mother and child. A child who is not breast-fed may receive less attention from and stimulation by his or her mother. Prevention of HIV transmission, including through breast-feeding, should be part of a comprehensive approach both to HIV prevention and care and to antenatal, perinatal and postnatal care and support. Policies should be made with the best interests in mind of the mother and baby as a pair.

The best way to prevent HIV transmission through breast-feeding is to prevent women from becoming infected in the first place. Develop and promote voluntary and confidential counselling and HIV testing services which are committed to informed consent and protection of confidentiality. A policy on infant feeding and HIV that is based on meeting the needs of Individual mothers and infants, requires that women know their HIV status. Improving access to counselling and testing for all women and their partners in antenatal care, family planning and all other appropriate points in the health service is necessary in order to implement Interventions to reduce MTCT, such as infant feeding options and antiretroviral drug treatment. Strengthen antenatal care services and encourage increased attendance so that they can provide information about prevention of HIV infection, HIV counselling and testing, offer Interventions to reduce MTCT, and refer HIV-positive women for infant feeding counselling, follow-up care and social support if needed. These should be provided in addition to the basic minimum package of antenatal care.

Some guidelines for prevention of HIV infection in women are the following.

— Educate the general public about how to avoid HIV infection. It must not be forgotten that the source of the woman's infection is usually her mate partner and father of the child.

— Develop policies and programmes to reduce girls' and women's vulnerability to HIV infection, especially their social and economic vulnerability, through improving their status in society.

— Target specifically the adolescent population for education about safe and responsible sexual behaviour.

— Ensure that couples have access to condoms so that they can act on their knowledge of safer sex.

— Provide information about MTCT, the importance of avoiding infection, and the advisability of practising safe sex during pregnancy and after giving birth as part of routine health education for men and women. programmes.

— Provide timely diagnosis and appropriate care for sexually transmitted diseases (STDs) including treatment for sexual partners, since STDs increase the risk of HIV transmission.

— Ensure that medical and surgical procedures such as injections and operations are performed with property sterilised instruments, and ensure safe blood transfusion services including screening of blood for transfusion.

Possible interventions to reduce the risk of MTCT by women who have been diagnosed HIV-infected include:

— *antiretroviral therapy (ARV)*: It is important to note that the efficacy of ARV has been proven when infants are not breast-fed but the efficacy when infants are not breast-fed but the efficacy when infants are breast-fed is currently unknown.

— *Modifications of obstetric care*: Including restricted use of invasive procedures to reduce the exposure of the infant to the blood of the infected mother. These measures can be implemented for all women, whatever their HIV status, and thus even before counselling and testing services are widely available.

— *Avoidance of breast-feeding*: Women need counselling about infant feeding options and support for their decision. They may need help with alternative feeding methods if they choose not to breast-feed.

Other possible interventions being studied and which may be beneficial for HIV-infected and HIV-uninfected mothers include:

— vitamin A supplements in areas where deficiency is prevalent

— cleansing of the birth canal during labour and delivery with a solution of the microbicide.

Consider infant feeding as part of a continuum of care and support services for women living with HIV and ensure that HIV positive women and their families have access to comprehensive health care including follow-up and social support. Protect, promote and support breast-feeding as the best infant feeding choice for uninfected women and women whose HIV status is not known. Breast-feeding remains the best source of nutrition for the great majority of infants.

In formulating policies to prevent HIV transmission through breast-feeding, care should be taken also to prevent the 'spillover effect', in which fear of HIV infection undermines the commitment to breast-feed even among women who are not infected, and undermines, too, support for breast-feeding by health systems and policies. Prevent commercial pressures for artificial feeding. All parents have a right to protection from promotion of breast-milk substitutes and feeding, bottles and teats.

Manufactures and distributors of products which fall within the scope of the International Code of Marketing of Breast-milk Substitutes should be reminded of their responsibilities under the Code and continue to take the necessary action to ensure that their conduct at every level conforms to its principles and aim. Governments should put specific emphasis on implementation of the Code in national legislation, regulations and other suitable measures to guarantee protection of all women including those mothers who choose not to breast-feed.

Preventing of MTCT requires strengthened maternity and family planning services, with increased access to antenatal care, counselling and testing for HIV, antiretroviral drugs and alternatives to breast-feeding. This is a complete package of care in which the supplies (test kits, drugs, breast-milk substitutes) are only one part. Provision of services for care and counselling, training of staff, and management of distribution are other vital components. The policy framework must recognize the wide diversity of personal situations and allow maximum flexibility in counselling individual women and families.

Setting priorities is an essential part of the policy-making process, and will require estimation of the costs of policy options, and of funds available to implement them.

A number of important points need to be considered when assessing the cost of measures to prevent MTCT of HIV. Items include:

i) *Organization of services*

- Strengthening of maternity services, especially increased antenatal care
- Allocation of staff time for counselling mothers about HIV Allocation of staff time for counselling mothers about infant feeding
- Arrangement of appropriate accommodation for counselling Provision of laboratory equipment to perform HIV tests. Provision of nutrition support and regular follow-up with growth monitoring for replacement-fed children for 2 years or more
- Increased access to family planning services for non-breast-feeding women
- Increased need for health care for non-breast-fed children (diarrhoea and other infections)

ii) *Training of staff*

- to counsel mothers on HIV; and on breast-feeding and replacement feeding
- to perform laboratory tests
- to provide ARV therapy

iii) *Provision of supplies*

- Laboratory equipment and supplies for HIV testing
- Breast-milk substitutes for HIV-positive women who choose not to breast-feed
- Antiretroviral (ARV) drugs, micronutrient supplements
- Additional costs to country
- Importation of supplies
- Distribution and management of supplies
- Monitoring of distribution
- Monitoring of child health indicators

iv) *Additional costs to families*

- Replacement feeding up to two years which is not subsidised
- Fuel, water for preparing feeds hygienically
- Increased health care costs

Care costs saved by averting HIV infections in children. The biggest expenditure is in setting up services (training, strengthening infrastructure). Thereafter, operating costs will be significantly tower. Some operating costs may be minimized by negotiation at national and international level, for example for the costs of tests kits, antiretroviral drugs and breast-milk substitutes.

Counselling programmes

To make informed decisions about how to feed their babies, mothers need to know whether or not they are HIV-Infected, and this requires that voluntary and confidential counselling and testing is provided and promoted. It is a fundamental principle that testing be voluntary and carried out with informed consent. Testing a pregnant or lactating woman without her full consent is unacceptable and a violation of human rights. Moreover, it is likely to deter women from seeking professional care through fear of disclosure and discrimination.

Testing must always be accompanied by pre-test and post-test counselling. Counselling is a dialogue, which alms to enable an individual to take decisions and find realistic ways of coping. Counselling is not the same as giving advice or telling people what they should do.

Counselling and testing must be confidential. Confidentiality is a right. Breaking confidentiality can expose an individual to discrimination. Promoting shared confidentiality means encouraging an individual to identify others whom they can trust such as their partner, a friend or health worker.

The ultimate goal is to provide widely available counselling and testing for the whole population. In the context of MTCT, it is particularly important that counselling and testing services are available for women of child-bearing age and their partners. It is recommended that services for women also involve partners when the woman so chooses, and that it be a duty of staff to encourage and facilitate this process.

Counselling is an intensive, skilled and time-consuming process that must answer a range of client needs. Every client must receive pre- and post-test counselling, and those who are HIV-positive are likely to require further counselling and support. In the case of pregnant and postpartum women this will include counselling and support about breast-feeding and replacement feeding.

The type of test to use. The most commonly used

type of antibody test is the ELISA (enzyme-linked immunosorbent assay). ELISA testing requires skilled technical staff, well-maintained equipment and a steady power supply. The price of ELISA and other screening tests ranges from around US$0.45 to $2.00. Rapid and simple antibody tests do not need such specialised equipment or staff but can equal the performance of ELISA. The result is usually available in a few hours, so it may be possible to give a person her result on the same day. However, 'same day results' tests may not be adequate where women need more time to cope fully with learning about their result. These tests are appropriate for use in small laboratories and in emergency testing, but they may be more expensive than ELISA.

Initial positive results for individual diagnosis must always be confirmed using a supplemental test, usually another type of ELISA, or a different kind of test (Western Blot], and/or a simple or rapid assay.

When children born to women living with HIV can be ensured uninterrupted access to nutritionally adequate breast-milk substitutes that are safely prepared and fed to them, they are at less risk of illness and death if they are not breast-fed. However, when these conditions are not fulfilled, in particular in an environment where infectious diseases and malnutrition are the primary causes of death during infancy, artificial feeding substantially increases children's risk of illness and death.'

In most countries, policy must cover a range of socioeconomic conditions, and the aim should be to promote and protect breast-feeding for the majority of Women while offering as much choice as possible to women who are HIV positive, enabling them to decide what is most appropriate for their circumstances and supporting them in their choice.

Replacement feeding

Using a specific term for feeding a child in the absence of breast milk is helpful to distinguish it from complementary feeding or various forms of artificial feeding which may be given in addition to breast milk. Support for adequate replacement feeding is needed throughout the period for which breast milk is recommended, and during which a child is at greatest risk of malnutrition: that is the first two years of life.

From birth to six months of age: An infant needs 150 ml milk per kg body weight per day. The milk should be prepared with careful attention to hygiene: this requires clean water to prepare the feed, and fuel to boil water, milk and utensils to kill microorganisms. Options include: Commercial infant formula, which is designed to meet the nutritional needs of an infant for the first four to six months of life. It may be made from cow's milk or vegetable products such as soy protein or a mixture of these. While important differences remain, these are the closest in composition to breast milk, and are usually adequately fortified with micronutrients including iron. The most widely available are in powdered form to be prepared by mixing with water. Feeding an infant for 6 months requires 40 × 500g tins (44 × 450g tins). Liquid ready-to-feed preparations are also available in some settings, but may be more expensive. Home-prepared formula, which can be made from animal milks, typically from cows, goats, buffaloes or sheep. The composition of animal milks is different from that of human milk, and they may provide insufficient micronutrients, especially iron, zinc, vitamin A,C and folic acid. It is best if they are modified for infants.

From six months to two years: Replacement feeding for a non-breast-fed infant should preferably continue to include a suitable breast-milk substitute and complementary foods made from appropriately prepared and nutrient-enriched family foods given three times a day. If suitable breast-milk substitutes are not available, replacement feeding should be with appropriately prepared and further enriched family foods given five times a day. If possible, other milk products such as unmodified animal milk, dried skimmed milk, or yoghurt should be included as a source of protein and calcium; other animal products such as meat, liver and fish should be given as a source of iron and zinc; and fruit and vegetables to provide vitamins, especially vitamins A and C. Micronutrient supplements should be given if available.

HIV-positive mothers who choose to breast-feed should consider this possibility as soon as they can provide adequate replacement feeds. No specific time is recommended. Expressing and heat treating breast milk. A mother can express her milk and either pasteurise it (heat to 62.5°C for 30 minutes) or boil it briefly and cool it. This kills the HIV virus. Mothers need to be highly motivated to feed this way over the long term at home. It may be more feasible in a hospital setting for sick and low-birth-weight infants who are at greater risk from artificial feeding and who may otherwise require special types of formula.

In some settings, breast milk may be available from milk banks. This may be most useful for sick and low-birth-weight babies. This can be considered an option if a milk bank is functioning according to recognised standards, and if donors are screened for HIV.

Wet-nursing in the family context is traditional in some cultures. There is a risk of HIV transmission to the infant if the wet-nurse is infected, and a possible risk of transmission to the wet-nurse if the infant is infected. If a family considers this option, both mother and wet-nurse should be fully informed about the risks. The wet-nurse should be offered counselling and testing, and be able to practise safe sex to remain HIV negative while breast-feeding the infant. The policy objective must be to minimise all infant feeding risks and to urgently expand access to adequate alternatives so that HIV-infected women have a range of choices. The policy should also stipulate what measures are being taken to make breast-milk substitutes available and affordable; to teach the safest means of feeding them to infants; and to provide the conditions which will diminish the risks of using them.

If the government offers free or subsidized breast-milk substitutes to some or all HIV-positive mothers who choose not to breast-feed, these mothers must be assured of breast-milk substitutes for at least six months. The calculation should be based on the assumption that one child will require approximately 20 kg of powdered infant formula or 92 litres of fresh milk for the first six months, and support for continued adequate replacement feeding up to two years of age, including some form of milk, if possible, up to at least one year. Locally produced fresh milk may be a more sustainable option than imported processed milks. Additional costs include micronutrient supplements and extra health care costs for no-breast-fed children. These are offset by reduced costs of treating fewer children with AIDS.

The risk of giving replacement feeds must be less than the risk of HIV transmission through breast-feeding, or there is no point in using them. Essential elements include knowledge and commitment on the part of care-givers, safe water, assured supplies of affordable fuel, easy access to quality health care for mothers and infants, and a good level of support from counsellors and/or social workers. Women choosing not to breast-feed will need extra support and counselling. Ideally this will be integrated into strengthened programmes for feeding and care of all infants. WHO and UNICEF recommend that infants be fed by cup rather than bottles and teats which are more difficult to use hygienically.

A policy recommendation that HIV-infected mothers be counselled about considering not breast-feeding can have major implications for birth-spacing. HIV-infected mothers who do not breast-feed are deprived of protection from lactational amenorrhea. If they do not use an appropriate form of family planning, they may have a shorter interval between births with adverse consequences for their own health. Ultimately, a larger number of potentially HIV-infected children will be born and will need to be cared for. Family planning information and services need to be made readily available to mothers and their partners.

If free or subsidised breast-milk substitutes are to be offered, they need to be distributed efficiently to the mothers who are eligible for them, but controlled to prevent encouraging use by mothers who are HIV negative or of unknown status. Possible ways to achieve this are by:

— central procurement of supplies, both to enable negotiation of favourable prices, and to facilitate control and monitoring of distribution

— giving breast-milk substitutes only to mothers who have had HIV counselling and testing and who know that they are positive

— allocation to local distribution points in appropriate quantities for the expected numbers of tested and HIV-infected women, to give an adequate amount without excess that may be used by other mothers

— careful storage to avoid loss and deterioration, and so that breast-feeding mothers do not see breast-milk substitutes displayed

— giving breast-milk substitutes through an accountable system of medical prescriptions or coupons, for example dispensed through pharmacies in the same way as medicines

— ensuring that an adequate supply will be made available for at least six months or for as long as the infant requires it

— ensuring that the provision of breast-milk substitutes is linked to follow-up visits, ideally at two- to four-week intervals.

HIV-negative women and those who do not know their status may decide not to breast-feed because of fears of HIV or misinformation. This would deprive their infants of the benefits of breast-feeding, and put them at risk of other infections and malnutrition. It is unlikely to be possible to give these mothers the extra support necessary to reduce the risks of artificial feeding. Possible ways to avoid spillover include:

— ensuring that health education programmes continue to emphasise the value of breast-feeding and the risks of artificial feeding. Information about MTCT should be given in a way that does not frighten mothers who are HIV negative or of unknown status, and lead them to avoid breast-feeding unnecessarily

— strengthening the Baby-friendly Hospital Initiative (BFHI), and ensuring that all health facilities implement practices to support breast-feeding, consistent with the 'Ten Steps to Successful Breast-feeding' which form the foundation of the BFHI. If a mother is

HIV-positive, this should be accepted as a medical indication for her not breast-feeding her infant

— making breast-feeding counselling available for all mothers who choose to breast-feed, whatever their HIV status

— ensuring that all staff who counsel mothers about replacement feeding are trained in breast-feeding counselling

— ensuring that instructions about replacement feeding are given privately to HIV-positive mothers and their families

— taking measures to implement the International Code of Marketing of Breast-milk Substitutes and subsequent relevant World Health Assembly resolutions. Health care workers should know about their responsibilities under the Code and apply them in their work

— arranging for breast-milk substitutes for HIV-positive mothers to be in generic, non-brand packaging.

Information, Education and Communication (IEC) is a very important element in a comprehensive policy on infant feeding, both to raise public awareness of the issues, and to encourage broad public debate that is based on accurate information. IEC is essential, too, in ensuring that policies are known about, acted upon, and are effective. The acceptability of counselling and testing and alternative feeding practices may be very low because of fear of stigmatization and rejection by the family and community; IEC programmes are thus an important component in the effort to reduce discrimination against HIV-infected people. Decision-makers will need to:

— allocate resources

— stipulate who should be responsible for preparing information

— consider where and how should be delivered so that it serves the purpose of informing without undermining breast-feeding practice. Several populations could be targeted by specific programmes: women, the general population, the health workers in the public sector, but also the private sector and NGOs

— ensure that information on replacement feeding adheres to the principles and aim of the International Code of Marketing of Breast-milk Substitutes

— ensure that advocacy for counselling and testing includes health professionals at all levels of the system and that IEC campaigns are designed to stimulate public debate and raise awareness of the benefits of HIV testing.

The International Code of Marketing of Breast-milk Substitutes recognizes that the encouragement and protection of breast-feeding is an important part of the health, nutrition and other social measures required to promote healthy growth and development of infants and young children, and that breast-feeding is an important aspect of primary health care.

The Code was adopted in response to concerns that the inappropriate marketing of breast-milk substitutes and related products was contributing to unsuitable feeding practices that placed infant health at risk. The Code aims to prevent the promotion of breast-milk substitutes and related products to the general public or through the health care system. These Guidelines are intended to be applied in accordance with all provisions of the Code and subsequent relevant World Health Assembly resolutions.

The Code does recognise that there are exceptional situations when alternatives to breast-feeding are necessary. The present guidelines provide advice concerning such an exceptional situation. They address the pressing public health issue of how best to meet the nutritional requirements of infants of HIV-infected mothers.

The guidelines suggest ways in which decision-makers can ensure such infants have access to breast-milk substitutes. At the same time, again recognizing that breast-feeding remains the best way to feed the vast majority of infants, the guidelines suggest ways in which breast-milk substitutes that are intended for infants who are at risk of HIV infection through breast-feeding reach only these children in need. Resolution WHA 47.5, paragraph 2(2) helps to ensure that the aforementioned conditions are satisfied by urging Member States 'to ensure that there are no donations of free or subsidized supplies of breast-milk substitutes and other products covered by the International Code of Marketing of Breast-milk Substitutes in any part of the health care system'.

In other words, Members States are urged to take measures to ensure that there is no donation of supplies of breast-milk substitutes from manufacturers or distributors in maternity and paediatric wards, MCH and family planning clinics, private doctor's offices and child-care institutions. However, the competent national authorities may wish to consider negotiating prices with manufacturers and making breast-milk substitutes available at a subsidized price or free of charge, for use by infants of mothers Living with HIV. It is recommended that this be done in a manner that:

— a long-term, reliable supply of suitable breast-milk substitutes and a dependable system for their distribution should be identified and secured

— does not create dependency on donated or Low-cost supplies of breast-milk substitutes

— such an arrangement is subject to the good will and generosity of the donor. If the donation ceases there may be no system in place to make breast-milk substitutes available to the infants who need them

— does not undermine breast-feeding for the majority of infants who would benefit from it

— does not have the effect of promoting breast-milk substitutes to the general public or the health care system

— assures individual infants sufficient quantities for as Long as they need them.

Where the health care or other competent authorities wish to make subsidized breast-milk substitutes available, these should, as a rule, be purchased through normal procurement channels. This ensures that they are made available only to infants that need to be fed artificially. Infants of mothers who have tested positive for the HIV virus fall into this category. This helps prevent the 'spillover effect' to infants who would otherwise benefit from breast-feeding. It is recommended that the following considerations be taken into account in organizing a distribution system.

— On average, forty 500g tins of commercial infant formula will be required during the first six months of the infant's Life. Quantities of free or subsidized breast-milk substitutes should be made available at a local, decentralized level to avoid the need for frequent trips to a distant distribution point.

— The receipt of free or subsidized breast-milk substitutes is Likely to become associated with HIV infection, and care is therefore needed to protect the anonymity of those receiving them to prevent potential stigmatization.

— A general reduction in the wholesale price of breast-milk substitutes by manufacturers as a part of a pricing policy intended to provide products at tow prices on a Long-term basis is permitted.

In the area of professional education and training, decision-makers need to consider:

— what staff are available who have already been trained in HIV counselling, laboratory testing and infant feeding, including the BFHI and breast-feeding counselling?

— who will be responsible for infant feeding counselling and what new staffing arrangements might be required?

— how many more staff with skills in breast-feeding and replacement feeding will be required? How will they be trained? By whom?

— what extra knowledge and skills will general health workers need, in both HIV and infant feeding, to refer families appropriately, and to give on-going support? Who will train them?

— what modifications or additions to the curricula for professional training will be required?

— what resources will it be necessary to allocate?

An IEC campaign aimed at encouraging awareness

and public debate about HIV and infant feeding issues should have the following aims:

— to move beyond simple messages of prevention that tend to reinforce the image of HIV/AIDS as a 'no hope' disease

— to counter denial of the existence or threat of HIV, and prejudice and discrimination against those infected

— to give the facts about mother-to-child transmission of HIV, including the availability of preventive interventions

— to reinforce messages about the value and importance of breast-feeding by women not known to be HIV-positive

— to reinforce messages about the benefits of adequate antenatal care

— to give the facts about treatment options for people with HIV/AIDS, and practical information about where to go for care, support and counselling

— to inform people about the benefits of counselling and testing, and to give them practical information about where services are available and how to use them, and to stimulate a public debate about testing

— to create awareness of the existence of relevant policies

— to reinforce messages about the benefits of family planning and contraception.

Decision-makers will need a thorough understanding of the situation regarding HIV/AIDS locally in order to formulate appropriate and effective policies. Organising a national workshop on the issue is a very useful way of gathering information and of involving a wide range of interested parties. Such an exercise may also be an effective way of encouraging cooperation and reducing tension around these very sensitive issues. Information needed to develop sound policies includes:

— identification of interested parties and key players—such as breast-feeding experts and NGOs, health care workers from baby-friendly hospitals, infant food producers including the dairy industry, paediatricians, nutritionists, those working in the field of HIV/AIDS, logistics experts —and the roles they could play in implementing policy. Manufacturers and distributors of products for infant feeding should not determine policy but may have a role in its effective application

— estimation of the numbers of mothers and infants likely to be affected; based on HIV prevalence, population and fertility

— assessment of the extent to which people infected with HIV arc stigmatised, and the possible social and cultural barriers to counselling and testing and replacement feeding

— assessment of attendance for antenatal care, family planning and related services - these provide opportunities to offer counselling and testing to prospective parents

— how many hospitals are baby-friendly? Can they be involved in the introduction of HIV counselling and testing and counselling about replacement feeding?

— availability of voluntary and confidential counselling and testing for HIV

— review of existing child feeding practices including:

  — breast-feeding rates

  — availability and costs (in relation to family incomes) of replacement feeds and micronutrient supplementation

  — morbidity and mortality associated with artificial feeding

  — average families' access to safe water, sanitation and fuel - and the feasibility of preparing replacement feeds safely

  — estimation of the amount of breast-milk substitutes needed by HIV-positive mothers, based on local HIV prevalence, fertility rates, and expected acceptability of HIV testing

  — availability of funding. Rather than diverting resources from other mother and child health programmes, decision-makers should use the opportunity of integrating these new tasks (HIV counselling and testing, counselling about infant feeding for HIV-Infected mothers) to strengthen basic maternity care, breast-feeding support, child care, family planning services and support services for HIV-Infected individuals.

After assessing the situation, priority tasks for implementing policy on HIV and infant feeding are:

— develop voluntary and confidential counselling and testing set-vices for HIV that arc integrated into the maternal child health services

— develop guidelines on infant feeding for different personnel—such as obstetricians, paediatricians, nutritionists, maternity nurses, counsellors. These guidelines should identify specifically who will be responsible for educating women about the proper use of breast-milk substitutes, and the level of support for infant feeding that HIV-positive women should receive, including follow-up and growth monitoring for at least two years

— develop training programmes and training materials. The priority areas should be counselling about breast-feeding and replacement feeding, management of breast-milk substitutes, counselling and support of HIV-infected women, food hygiene

— plan and develop a counselling service for breast-feeding and replacement feeding that is integrated into maternal and child health services. Consider staffing requirements

— assess additional family planning and contraceptive needs for non-breast-feeding women, and ensure that supplies of and access to condoms is adequate

— allocate responsibilities for the various tasks to be performed and draw up time-lines for the Implementation of the policy. Breast-feeding and HIV/AIDS NGOs should be involved

— develop and disseminate messages for the general public.

If it is decided to provide free or subsidised supplies of breast-milk substitutes to eligible mothers:

— organise the procurement of breast-milk substitutes

— arrange their distribution to the health services or other distribution points

— set up mechanisms for controlling and monitoring their distribution.

Monitoring health outcomes including HIV status and growth in children of HIV-positive mothers who breast-feed or feed artificially, as well as health effects in other children and family members of women who artificially feed, will help in refining national policies and counselling practices. It will also be necessary to monitor the distribution and correct use of breast-milk substitutes. Monitoring breast-feeding rates in HIV-negative women will indicate whether 'spillover' is occurring—that is whether breast-feeding practice is being undermined by anxiety over HIV and easier access generally to breast-milk substitutes - and enable steps to be taken to counter spillover, if necessary.

Planners and administrators need to identify which indicators to use and decide how frequently monitoring and evaluation will be done; who will be responsible, and the mechanisms for reporting and follow-up. Interested parties and key players such as NGOs may have a useful role to play.

The baseline studies or situation analysis on which a policy or programme is based offer useful yardsticks against which to measure change and progress. Suggested indicators are those included in 'Indicators for assessing breast-feeding practices', which includes the exclusive breast-feeding rate, timely complementary feeding rate, continued breast-feeding rate, and bottle-feeding rate.

The number of infants born with HIV infection is growing every day. The AIDS pandemic represents a tragic setback in the progress made on child welfare and survival. Given the vital importance of breast milk and breast-feeding for child health, the increasing prevalence of HIV infection around the world, and the evidence of a risk of HIV transmission through breast-feeding, it is now crucial that policies be developed on HIV infection and infant feeding.

All women and men, irrespective of their HIV status, have the right to determine the course of their reproductive life and health, and to have access to information and services that allow them to protect their own and their family's health. Where the welfare of children is concerned, decisions should be made that are in keeping with children's best interests.

Majority of HIV-infected children have been infected through their mothers, most of whom have been infected through unprotected heterosexual intercourse. High priority therefore, now and in the long term, should be given to policies and programmes aimed at reducing women's vulnerability to HIV infection, especially their social and economic vulnerability—through improving their status in society. Immediate practical measures should include ensuring access to information about HIV/AIDS and its prevention, promotion of safer sex including the use of condoms, and adequate treatment of sexually transmitted diseases which significantly increase the risk of HIV transmission.

Breast-feeding provides substantial benefits to both children and mothers. It significantly improves child survival by protecting against diarrhoeal diseases, pneumonia and other potentially fatal infections, while it enhances quality of life through its nutritional and psychosocial benefits. In contrast, artificial feeding Increases risks to child health and contributes to child mortality.

Breast-feeding contributes to maternal health in various ways including prolonging the interval between births, and helping to protect against ovarian and breast cancers. However, there is evidence that

HIV—the virus that causes AIDS—can be transmitted through breast-feeding. Various studies conducted to date indicate that between one-quarter and one-third of infants born worldwide to women infected with HIV become infected with the virus themselves.

While in most cases transmission occurs during late pregnancy and delivery, preliminary studies indicate that more than one-third of these infected infants are infected through breast-feeding. These studies suggest an average risk for HIV transmission through breast-feeding of one in seven children born to, and breast-fed by, a woman living with HIV (i.e. infected with HIV).

Additional data are needed to identify precisely the timing of transmission through breast-feeding (in order to provide mothers living with HIV with better information about the risks and benefits of early weaning), to quantify the risk attributable to breast-feeding, and to determine the associated risk factors. Studies are also needed to access other interventions for reducing mother-to-child transmission of HIV infection.

Elements for establishing a policy on infant feeding

Supporting breast-feeding: As a general principle, in all populations, irrespective of HIV infection rates, breast-feeding should continue to be protected, promoted and supported.

Improving access to HIV—counselling and testing: Access to voluntary and confidential HIV counselling and testing should be facilitated for women and men of reproductive age, in part by ensuring a supportive environment that encourages individuals to be informed and counselled about their HIV status rather than one that discourages them out of fear of discrimination or stigmatization. As part of the counselling process, women and men of reproductive age should be informed of the implications of their HIV status for the health and welfare of their children. Counselling for women who are aware of their HIV status should include the best available information on the benefits of breast-feeding, on the risk of HIV transmission through breast-feeding, and on the risks and possible advantages associated with other methods of infant feeding.

Ensuring informed choice: Because both parents have a responsibility for the health and welfare of their children, and because the infant feeding method chosen has health and financial implications for the entire family, mothers and fathers should be encouraged to reach a decision together on this matter.

However, it is mothers who are in the best position to decide whether to breast-feed, particularly when they alone may know their HIV status and wish to exercise their right to keep that information confidential. It is therefore important that women be empowered to make fully informed decisions about infant feeding, and that they be suitably supported in carrying them out. This should include efforts to promote a hygienic environment, essentially clean water and sanitation, that will minimize health risks when a breast-milk substitute is used.

When children born to women living with HIV can be ensured uninterrupted access to nutritionally adequate breast-milk substitutes that are safely prepared and fed to them, they arc at less risk of illness and death if they are not breast-fed. However, when these conditions are not fulfilled, in particular in an environment where infectious diseases and malnutrition are the primary causes of death during infancy, artificial feeding substantially increases children's risk of illness and death.

Preventing commercial pressures for artificial feeding: Manufacturers and distributors of products which fall within the scope of the International Code of Marketing of Breast-milk Substitutes (1981) should be reminded of their responsibilities under the Code and continue to take the necessary action to ensure that their conduct at every level conforms to the principles and aim of the Code.

International code for marketing of breast-milk substitutes

PREAMBLE The Member States of the World Health Organization:

AFFIRMING the right of every child and every lactating woman to be adequately nourished as a means of attaining and maintaining health;

RECOGNIZING that infant malnutrition is part of the wider problems of lack of education, poverty and social injustice;

RECOGNIZING that the health of infants and young children cannot be isolated from the health and nutrition of women, their socioeconomic status and their roles as mothers;

CONSCIOUS that breast-feeding is an unequalled, way of providing ideal food, for the healthy growth and development of infants; that it forms a unique, biological and emotional basis for the health of both mother and child; that the anti-infective properties of breast milk, help to protect infants against disease; and that there is an important relationship between breast-feeding and child-spacing;

RECOGNIZING that the encouragement and protection of breast-feeding is an important, part of the health, nutrition and other social measures required to promote healthy growth and development of infants and young children; and that breast-feeding is an important, aspect Of primary health care;

CONSIDERING that when mothers do not breast-feed, or only do so partially, there is a legitimate market, for infant formula and for suitable ingredients from which to prepare it; that all these products should accordingly be made accessible to those who need them, through commercial or non-commercial distribution systems; and that they should not be marketed or distributed in ways that interfere with the protection and promotion of breast-feeding;

RECOGNIZING further that inappropriate infant feeding practices, lead to infant malnutrition, morbidity and mortality in all countries, and that improper practices in the marketing of breast-milk substitutes and related products, can contribute to these major public health problems;

CONVINCED that it is important, for infants to receive appropriate complementary foods, usually when the infant reaches four to six months of age, and that every effort should be made to use locally, available foods; and convinced, nevertheless, that such complementary foods should not be used as breast-milk substitutes;

APPRECIATING that there are a number of social and economic factors, affecting breast-feeding, and that, accordingly, governments should develop social support systems, to protect, facilitate and encourage it, and that they should create an environment that fosters breast-feeding, provides appropriate family and community support, and protects mothers, from factors that inhibit breast-feeding;

AFFIRMING that health care systems, and the health professionals and other health workers serving in them, have an essential role, to play in guiding infant feeding practices, encouraging and facilitating breast-feeding, and providing objective and consistent advice, to mothers and families about the superior value of breast-feeding, or, where needed, on the proper use of infant formula, whether manufactured industrially or home-prepared;

AFFIRMING further that educational systems and other social services should be involved in the protection and promotion of breast-feeding, and in the appropriate use of complementary foods;

AWARE that families, communities, women's organizations and other non-governmental organizations have a special role to play in the protection and promotion of breast-feeding and in ensuring the support needed by pregnant women and mothers of infants and young children, whether breast-feeding or not;

AFFIRMING the need for governments, organizations of the United Nations system, non-governmental organizations, experts in various related disciplines, consumer groups and industry to cooperate in activities aimed at the improvement of maternal, infant and young child health and nutrition;

RECOGNIZING that governments should undertake a variety of health, nutrition and other social measures to promote healthy growth and development of infants and young children, and that this Code concerns only one aspect of these measures;

CONSIDERING that manufacturers and distributors of breast-milk substitutes have an important and constructive role to play in relation to breast feeding, and in the promotion Of the aim of this Code and its proper implementation;

AFFIRMING that governments are called upon to take action appropriate to their social and legislative framework and their overall development objectives to give effect to the principles and aim of this Code, including the enactment of legislation, regulations or other suitable measures;

BELIEVING that, in the light of the foregoing considerations, and in view of the vulnerability of infants in the early months of life and the risks involved in inappropriate feeding practices, including the unnecessary and improper use of breast-milk substitutes, the marketing of breast-milk substitutes requires special treatment, which makes usual marketing practices unsuitable, for these products;

THEREFORE: The Member States hereby agree the following articles which are recommended as a basis for action.

Article 1: Aim of the Code

The aim of this Code is to contribute to the provision of safe and adequate nutrition for infants, by the protection and promotion of breast-feeding, and by ensuring the proper use of breast-milk substitutes, when these are necessary, on the basis of adequate information and through appropriate marketing and distribution.

Article 2: Scope of the Code

The Code applies to the marketing, and practices related thereto, of the following products: breast-milk substitutes, including infant formula; other milk products, foods and beverages, including bottle-fed complementary foods, when marketed or otherwise represented to be suitable, with or without modification, for use as a partial or total replacement of breast milk-, feeding bottles, and teats. It also applies to their quality and availability, and to information concerning their use.

Article 3: Definitions

For the purposes of this Code: Breast-milk substitute means any food being marketed or otherwise represented as a partial or total replacement for breast milk, whether or not suitable for that purpose.

Complementary food means any food, whether manufactured or locally prepared, suitable as a complement to breast milk or to infant formula, when either becomes insufficient to satisfy the nutritional requirements of the infant. Such food is also commonly called 'weaning food' or 'breast-milk supplement'.

Container means any form of packaging of products for sale as a normal retail unit, including wrappers.

Distributor means a person, corporation or any other entity in the public or private sector engaged in the business (whether directly or indirectly) of marketing at the wholesale or retail level a product within the scope of this Code. A 'primary distributor' is a manufacturer's sales agent, representative, national distributor or broker.

Health care system means governmental, nongovernmental or private institutions or organizations engaged, directly or indirectly, in health care for mothers, infants and pregnant women; and nurseries or child-care institutions. It also includes health workers in private practice. For the purposes of this Code, the health care system does not include pharmacies or other established sales outlets.

Health worker means a person working in a component of such a health care system, whether professional or non-professional, including voluntary, unpaid workers.

Infant formula means a breast-milk substitute formulated industrially in accordance with applicable Codex Alimentarius standards, to satisfy the normal nutritional requirements of infants up to between four and six months of age, and adapted to their physiological characteristics. Infant formula may also be prepared at home, in which case It is described as 'home-prepared'.

Label means any tag, brand, mark, pictorial or other descriptive matter, written, printed, stencilled, marked, embossed or impressed on, or attached to, a container (see above) of any products within the scope of this Code.

Manufacturer means a corporation or other entity in the public or private sector engaged in the business or function (whether directly or through an agent or through an entity controlled by or under contract with it) of manufacturing a product within the scope of this Code.

Marketing means product promotion, distribution, selling, advertising, product public relations, and information services.

Marketing personnel means any persons whose functions involve the marketing of a product or products coming within the scope of this Code. Samples means single or small quantities of a product provided without cost. Supplies means quantities of a product provided for use over an extended period, free or at a low price, for social purposes, including those provided to families in need.

Article 4: Information and education

4.1 Governments, should have the responsibility to ensure that objective and consistent information, is provided on infant and young child feeding for use by families and those involved in the field of infant and young child nutrition. This responsibility should cover either the planning, provision, design and dissemination of information or their control.

4.2 Informational and educational materials, whether written, audio or visual, dealing with the feeding of infants and intended to reach pregnant women and mothers of infants and young children, should include Clear, information on all, the following points: (a) the benefits and superiority of breast-feeding; (b) maternal nutrition, and the preparation for and maintenance of breast-feeding; (c) the negative effect, on breast-feeding of introducing partial bottle-feeding; (d) the difficulty of reversing the decision, not to breast-feed; and, (e) where needed, the proper use of infant formula, whether manufactured industrially or home-prepared. When, such materials contain information about the use of infant formula, they should include the social and financial implications, of its use; the health hazards, of inappropriate foods or feeding methods; and, in particular, the health hazards of unnecessary or improper use, of infant formula and other breast-milk substitutes. Such materials should not use any pictures or text which may idealize, the use of breast-milk substitutes.

4.3 Donations of informational or educational equipment or materials by manufacturers or distributors should be made only at the request and with the written approval, of the appropriate government authority or within guidelines given by governments for this purpose. Such equipment or materials may bear the donating company's name or logo, but should not refer to a proprietary product that is within the scope of this Code, and should be distributed only through the health care system.

Article 5: The general public and mothers

5.1 There should be no advertising or other form of promotion to the general public of products within the scope of this Code.

5.2 Manufacturers and distributors should not provide, directly or indirectly, to pregnant women, mothers or members of their families, samples of products within the scope of this Code.

5.3 In conformity with paragraphs 1 and 2 of this Article, there should be no point-of-sale advertising, giving of samples, or any other promotion device to induce sales directly to the consumer at the retail level, such as special displays, discount coupons, premiums, special sales, loss-leaders and tie-in sales, for products within the scope of this Code. This provision should not restrict the establishment of pricing policies and practices intended to provide products at lower prices on a long-term basis.

5.4 Manufacturers and distributors should not distribute, to pregnant women or mothers of infants and young children any gifts of articles or utensils which may promote the use of breast-milk substitutes or bottle-feeding.

5.5 Marketing personnel, in their business capacity, should not seek direct or indirect contact, of any kind with pregnant women or with mothers, of infants and young children.

Article 6: Health care systems

6.1 The health authorities in Member States should take appropriate measures to encourage and protect breast-feeding and promote the principles of this Code, and should give appropriate information and advice to health workers, in regard to their responsibilities, including the information specified in Article 4.2.

6.2 No facility of a health care system should be used for the purpose of promoting infant formula or other products within the scope of this Code. This Code does not, however, preclude the dissemination of information to health professionals as provided in Article 7.2.

6.3 Facilities of health care systems should not be used for the display of products, within the scope of this Code, for placards or posters, concerning such products, or for the distribution of material, provided by a manufacturer or distributor other than that specified in Article 4.3.

6.4 The use by the health care system of professional service representatives', mothercraft nurses' or similar personnel, provided or paid for by manufacturers or distributors, should not be permitted.

6.5 Feeding with infant formula, whether manufactured or home-prepared, should be demonstrated only by health workers, or other community workers if necessary; and only to the mothers or family members who need to use it-, and the information given should include a clear explanation of the hazards of improper use

6.6 Donations or low-price sales to institutions or organizations of supplies of infant formula or other products within the scope of this Code, whether for use in the institution or for distribution outside them, may be made. Such supplies should only be used or distributed for infants who have to be fed on breast-milk substitutes. If these supplies are distributed for use outside the institutions, this should be done only by the institutions or organizations concerned. Such donations or low-priced sales should not be used by manufacturers or distributors as a sales inducement.

6.7 Where donated supplies of infant formula or other products within the scope of this Code are distributed outside an institution, the institution or organization should take steps to ensure that supplies can be continued as long as the infants concerned need them. Donors, as well as institutions or organizations concerned, should bear in mind this responsibility.

6.8 Equipment and materials, in addition to those referred to in Article 4.3, donated to a health care system may bear a company's name or logo, but should not refer to any proprietary product, within the scope of this Code.

Article 7: Health workers

7.1 Health workers should encourage and protect breast-feeding; and those who are concerned in particular with maternal and infant nutrition should make themselves familiar with their responsibilities under this Code, including the information specified in Article 4.2.

7.2 Information provided, by manufacturers and distributors to health professionals, regarding products within the scope of this Code should be restricted to scientific and factual matters, and such information should not imply or create a belief that bottle feeding is equivalent or superior to breast-feeding. It should also include the information specified in Article 4.2.

7.3 No financial or material inducements, to promote products within the scope of this Code should be offered by manufacturers or distributors to health workers or members of their families, nor should these be accepted by health workers or members of their families.

7.4 Samples, of infant formula or other products within the scope of this Code, or of equipment or utensils for their preparation or use, should not be provided to health workers except when necessary for the purpose of professional evaluation or research, at the institutional level. Health workers should not give samples, of infant formula to pregnant women, mothers of infants and young children, or members of their families.

7.5 Manufacturers and distributors of products within the scope of this Code should disclose, to the institution to which a recipient health worker is affiliated any contribution, made to him or on his behalf for fellowships, study tours, research grants, attendance at professional conferences, or the like. Similar disclosures should be made by the recipient.

Article 8: Persons employed by manufacturers and distributors

8.1 In systems of sales incentives for sales personnel, the volume of sales, of products within the scope of this Code should not be included in the calculation of bonuses, nor should quotas be set specifically for sales, of these products. This should not be understood to prevent the payment of bonuses based on the overall sales by a company of other products marketed by it.

8.2 Personnel employed in marketing, products within the scope of this Code should not, as part of their Job responsibilities, perform education functions in relation to pregnant women or mothers of infant and young children. This should not be understood as preventing such personnel from being used for other functions by the health care system at the request and with the written approval of the appropriate authority of the government concerned.

Article 9: Labelling

9.1 Labels should be designed to provide the necessary information about the appropriate use of the product, and so as not to discourage breast-feeding.

9.2 Manufacturers and distributors of infant formula should ensure that each container has a clear, conspicuous, and easily readable and understandable message, printed on it, or on a label which cannot readily become separated from it, in an appropriate language, which includes all the following points:

a) the words 'Important Notice' or their equivalent;

b) a statement of the superiority of breast-feeding;

c) a statement that the product should be used only on the advice of a health worker as to the need for its use and the proper method of use;

d) instructions for appropriate preparation, and a warning against the health hazards of inappropriate preparation.

Neither the container nor the label should have pictures of infants, nor, should they have other pictures or text which may idealize the use of infant formula. They may, however, have graphics for easy identification of the product as a breast-milk substitute and for illustrating methods of preparation. The terms 'humanized', 'maternalized' or similar terms should not be used. Inserts giving additional information about the product and its proper use, subject to the above conditions, may be included in the package or retail unit. When labels give instructions for modifying a product into Infant formula, the above should apply.

9.3 Food products, within the scope of this Code, marketed for infant feeding, which do not meet all the requirements of an infant formula, but which can be modified to do so, should carry on the label a warning, that the unmodified product should not be the sole source of nourishment of an infant. Since sweetened condensed milk is not suitable for infant feeding, nor for use as a main ingredient of infant formula, its label should not contain purported instructions on how to modify it for that purpose.

9.4 The label of food products within the scope of this Code should also state all the following points:

a) the ingredients used;

b) the composition/analysis of the product;

c) the storage conditions required; and

d) the batch number, and the date before which the product is to be consumed, taking into account the climatic and storage conditions of the country concerned.

Article 10: Quality

10.1 The quality of products is an essential element for the protection of the health of infants and therefore should be of a high recognized standard.

10.2 Food products within the scope of this Code should, when sold or otherwise distributed, meet applicable standards recommended by the Codex Alimentarius Commission, and also the Codex Code of Hygienic Practice for Foods for Infants and Children.

Article 11: Implementation and monitoring

11.1 Governments should take action, to give effect to the principles and aim of this code, as appropriate to their social and legislative framework, including the adoption of national legislation, regulations or other suitable measures. For this purpose, governments should seek, when necessary, the cooperation of

WHO, UNICEF and other agencies of the United Nations system. National policies and measures, including laws and regulations, which are adopted to give effect to the principles and aim of this Code should be publicly stated, and should apply on the same basis to all those involved in the manufacture and marketing of products within the scope of this Code.

11.2 Monitoring the application of this Code lies with governments, acting individually, and collectively through the World Health Organization as provided in paragraphs 6 and 7 of this Article. The manufacturers and distributors, of products within the scope of this Code, and appropriate nongovernmental organizations, professional groups, and consumer organizations should collaborate with governments to this end.

11.3 Independently of any other measures taken for implementation of this Code, manufacturers and distributors, of products within the scope of this Code should regard themselves as responsible for monitoring their marketing practices, according to the principles and aim of this Code, and for taking steps to ensure that their conduct at every level conforms to them.

11.4 Non-governmental organizations, professional groups, institutions and individuals concerned should have the responsibility of drawing the attention of manufacturers or distributors to activities which are incompatible, with the principles and aim of this Code, so that appropriate action can be taken. The appropriate governmental authority should also be informed.

11.5 Manufacturers and primary distributors of

products within the scope of this Code should apprise each member of their marketing personnel of the Code and of their responsibilities under it.

11.6 In accordance with Article 62 of the Constitution of the World Health Organization, Member States shall communicate annually to the Director-General information on action taken, to give effect to the principles and aim of this Code.

11.7 The Director-General shall report in even years to the World Health Assembly on the status of implementation of the Code; and shall, on request, provide technical support to Member States preparing national legislation or regulations, or taking other appropriate measures in implementation and furtherance of the principles and aim of this Code.

Infant and young child feeding

The Thirty-ninth World Health Assembly,

Recalling resolutions WHA27.43, WHA31.47, WHA33.32, WHA34.22, WHA35.26 and WHA37.30 which dealt with infant and young child feeding;

Having considered the progress and evaluation report on infant and young child nutrition;

Recognizing that the implementation of the International Code of Marketing of Breast-milk Substitutes is an important contribution to healthy infant and young child feeding in all countries;

Aware that today, five years after the adoption of the International Code, many Member States have made substantial efforts to implement it, but that many products unsuitable for infant feeding are nonetheless being promoted and used for this purpose; and that sustained and concerted efforts will therefore continue to be necessary to achieve full implementation of and compliance with the International Code as well as the cessation of the marketing of unsuitable products and the improper promotion of breast-milk substitutes;

Noting with great satisfaction the Guidelines concerning the main health and socioeconomic circumstances in which infants have to be fed on breast-milk substitutes,' in the context of Article 6, paragraph 6, of the International Code;

Noting further the statement in the Guidelines, paragraph 47: "Since the large majority of infants born in maternity wards and hospitals are full term, they require no nourishment other than colostrum during their first 24-48 hours of life - the amount of time often spent by a mother and her infant in such an institutional setting. Only small quantities of breast-milk substitutes are ordinarily required to meet the needs of a minority of infants in these facilities, and they should only be available in ways that do not interfere with the protection and promotion of breast-feeding for the majority.";

1. ENDORSES the report of the Director-General;

2. URGES Member States:

   (1) to implement the Code if they have not yet done so;

   (2) to ensure that the practices and procedures of their health care systems are consistent with the principles and aim of the International Code;

   (3) to make the fullest use of all concerned parties—health professional bodies,

nongovernmental organizations, consumer organizations, manufacturers and distributors - generally, in protecting and promoting breast-feeding and, specifically, in implementing the Code and monitoring its implementation and compliance with its provisions;

(4) to seek the cooperation of manufacturers and distributors of products within the scope of Article 2 of the Code, in providing all information considered necessary for monitoring the implementation of the Code;

(5) to provide the Director-General with complete and detailed information on the implementation of the Code;

(6) to ensure that the small amounts of breast-milk substitutes needed for the minority of infants who require them in maternity wards and hospitals are made available through the normal procurement channels and not through free or subsidized supplies;

3. Requests the Director-General:

(1) to propose a simplified and standardized form for use by Member States to facilitate the monitoring and evaluation by them of their implementation of the Code and reporting thereon to WHO, as well as the preparation by WHO of a consolidated report covering each of the articles of the Code;

(2) to specifically direct the attention of Member States and other interested parties to the following: (a) any food or drink given before complementary feeding is

nutritionally required may interfere with the initiation or maintenance of breast feeding and therefore should neither be promoted nor encouraged for use by infants during this period; (b) the practice being introduced in some countries of providing infants with specially formulated milks (so-called "follow-up" milks) is not necessary.

Infant and young child nutrition

The Forty-seventh World Health Assembly,

Having considered the report by the Director-General on infant and young child nutrition;

Recalling resolutions WHA33.32, WHA34.22, WHA35.26, WHA37.30, WHA39.28, WHA41.11, WHA43.3, WHA45.34 and WHA46.7 concerning infant and young child nutrition, appropriate feeding practices and related questions;

Reaffirming its support for all these resolutions and reiterating the recommendations to Member States contained therein;

Bearing in mind the superiority of breast-milk as the biological norm for the nourishment of infants, and that a deviation from this norm is associated with increased risks to the health of infants and mothers;

1. Thanks the Director-General for his report;
2. Urges Member States to take the following measures:
   (1) to promote sound infant and young child nutrition, in keeping with their commitment to the World Declaration and Plan of Action for Nutrition, through coherent effective intersectoral action, including:

(a) increasing awareness among health personnel, nongovernmental organizations, communities and the general public of the importance of breast-feeding and its superiority to any other infant feeding method;

(b) supporting mothers in their choice to breast-feed by removing obstacles and preventing interference that they may face in health services, the workplace, or the community;

(c) ensuring that all health personnel concerned are trained in appropriate infant and young child feeding practices, including the application of the principles laid down in the joint WHO/UNICEF statement on breast-feeding and the role of maternity services.

(d) fostering appropriate complementary feeding practices from the age of about six months, emphasizing continued breast-feeding and frequent feeding with safe and adequate amounts of local foods;

(2) to ensure that there are no donations of free or subsidized supplies of breast milk substitutes and other products covered by the International Code of Marketing of Breast-milk Substitutes in any part of the health care system;

(3) to exercise extreme caution when planning, implementing or supporting emergency relief operations, by protecting, promoting and supporting breast-feeding for infants.

and ensuring that donated supplies of breast-milk substitutes or other products covered by the scope of the International Code be given only if all the following conditions apply:

(a) infants have to be fed on breast-milk substitutes, as outlined in the guidelines concerning the main health and socioeconomic circumstances in which infants have to be fed on breast-milk substitutes.

(b) the supply is continued for as long as the infants concerned need it;

(c) the supply is not used as a sales inducement;

(4) to inform the labour sector, and employers' and workers' organizations, about the multiple benefits of breast-feeding for infants and mothers, and the implications for maternity protection in the workplace;

3. Requests the Director-General:

(1) to use his good offices for cooperation with all parties concerned in giving effect to this and related resolutions of the Health Assembly in their entirety;

(2) to complete development of a comprehensive global approach and programme of action to strengthen national capacities for improving infant and young child feeding practices; including the development of methods and criteria for national assessment of breast-feeding trends and practices;

(3) to support Member States, at their request, in monitoring infant and young child

feeding practices and trends in health facilities and households, in keeping with new standard breast-feeding indicators;

(4) to urge Member States to Join in the Baby-friendly Hospital Initiative and to support them, at their request, in implementing this Initiative, particularly in their efforts to improve educational curricula and in-service training for all health and administrative personnel concerned;

(5) to increase and strengthen support to Member States, at their request, in giving effect to the principles and aim of the International Code and all relevant resolutions, and to advise Member States on a framework which they may use in monitoring their application, as appropriate to national circumstances;

(6) to develop, in consultation with other concerned parties and as part of WHO's normative function, guiding principles for the use in emergency situations of breast-milk substitutes or other products covered by the International Code which the competent authorities in Member States may use, in the light of national circumstances, to ensure the optimal infant feeding conditions;

(7) to complete, in cooperation with selected research institutions, collection of revised reference data and the preparation of guidelines for their use and interpretation, so as to assess the growth of breast-fed infants;

(8) to seek additional technical and financial resources for intensifying WHO's support to Member States in infant feeding and in the implementation of the International Code and subsequent relevant resolutions.

Advances in knowledge and understanding of HIV have greatly increased the options for care of infected people and therefore the benefits to the individual of knowing his or her serostatus.

People who know they are HIV-Infected are likely to be motivated to look after their health, perhaps with behaviour and lifestyle changes, and to seek early medical attention for problems They can make informed decisions about sexual practices and child-bearing, mothers can make informed decisions about infant feeding, and about seeking care for sick children without delay.

Moreover, they can take steps to protect partners who may still be uninfected. In places where antiretroviral (ARV) therapy is available, only those women who know they are HIV-positive will have the opportunity to benefit from it. Those whose test result is negative should be counselled about how to protect themselves - and their children - from infection

Among the disadvantages is the possibility that knowledge of their status will expose infected people to stigmatization and discrimination, and perhaps even violence and abandonment. These remain serious problems in many places and need urgently to be addressed.

For example, instead of testing women alone as part of the package of maternity care, the policy should be to encourage testing of both partners, thus promoting Joint responsibility and decision-making regarding sexual behaviour, reproduction, and infant care. This is especially Important in societies where many of these decisions are traditionally taken by men.

Mandatory testing of pregnant women as a public health measure is a violation of human rights and is not acceptable. Guaranteeing confidentiality of test results, a fundamental principle of HIV testing, also helps to protect people from stigmatization. But in the long run, counselling and testing services themselves play an important part in dispelling prejudice and fear surrounding HIV/AIDS.

The more people who know their HIV status and share their knowledge with family and friends, the more public awareness grows that HIV infection is not automatically fatal nor a threat to casual contacts. Indeed, it spreads awareness that much can be done to prevent transmission of the virus and to enhance the survival and quality of life of people infected. Since the primary purpose of counselling and testing is to encourage informed decision-making and behaviour, it is very important that individuals have ready access to the services they need. These include : family planning services for those women or couples who wish to avoid or postpone pregnancy, or practice safe sex during pregnancy and lactation; mother and child health and other health care and support services for HIV-positive people with health problems and social and psychological needs.

Good links and efficient referral systems will encourage people to use counselling and testing services. What are the costs involved in counselling and testing? The biggest expenditure is in setting up services—especially in situations where the existing infrastructure of laboratories and health facilities needs adapting and strengthening and staff require extensive retraining in counselling.

Thereafter the main recurrent expenses are the test kits, staff salaries, information, education and communication (IEC) activities.

The risk of mother-to-child transmission of HIV can be reduced substantially if a woman known to be HIV-positive is given antiretroviral (ARV) therapy during pregnancy labour', and her infant is given ARV for the first six weeks of life and is not breast-fed by her.

The therapy was developed by French and American scientists who announced in 1994 the results of research with the antiretroviral drug zidovudine, or AZT.

They found that when AZT is given to HIV-positive women orally from the 14th week of pregnancy onwards and intravenously during labour, and to their infants for six weeks after birth, the risk of transmitting HIV from mother to child is reduced by nearly 70 per cent.

However, the regimen is costly and complicated to administer, and the impressive results may depend on complete avoidance of breast-feeding. Researchers in Thailand have reported in early 1998 that AZT taken by mouth twice daily from the 36th week of pregnancy until the onset of labour and during labour reduced the risk of mother-to-child transmission by approximately one half in their study subjects.

None of the infants was breast-fed, and the mothers were provided with infant formula by the research programme. The cost of the drugs for each mother/child pair in this programme was approximately US$50, compared with around US$1,000 for the regimen developed by the French and American teams. The efficacy of AZT in preventing HIV transmission to the child from an

HIV-positive mother who breast-feeds is currently not known.

AZT may provide some degree of protection, although probably less than the protection it provides to infants who are not breast-fed. Nevertheless, the greatest reduction in mother to child transmission of HIV is likely to occur when an integrated prevention programme is implemented which combines the provision of AZT and adequate alternatives to breast-feeding. In some countries, it may prove to be impractical to implement simultaneously access to AZT and access to adequate alternatives to breast-feeding. In these situations, the implementation of one prevention component should not be delayed until the other is feasible.

Furthermore, in societies where breast-feeding is the norm, a mother who does not breast-feed her baby may be marked out as HIV-infected and risk stigmatisation and possibly violence and rejection. In these circumstances, a therapy that Is contingent upon not breast-feeding will raise painful dilemmas for the individual mother and her counsellor.

If a woman chooses not to use both AZT and adequate alternatives to breast-feeding, she should still have access to the intervention of her choice and should be supported to carry out the use of this intervention safely and effectively. A key precondition of introducing ARV therapy is that counselling and testing services be in place and operating efficiently. It is also a prerequisite that women have access to good quality antenatal and postnatal services and give birth in a maternity ward or clinic, with professional assistance.

5

Social Impacts of AIDS

The greatest hope for combating HIV/AIDS in the foreseeable future is that of helping people to choose safer behaviour so that they will be less likely to contract and spread HIV.

The first aim should be to influence individual choices directly within the existing economic and social context by changing the costs and benefits of various types of behaviour, making safer behaviour a more attractive choice. However, individual behaviour is shaped and often constrained by the economic and social context; some individuals choices are very constrained.

A second, complementary approach is to change the economic and social conditions that make it difficult or impossible for some people to protect themselves from HIV. The benefits of this approach typically extend far beyond HIV prevention. It is therefore often difficult to assess the cost-effectiveness of measures to affect the economic and social environment, but they are likely to improve the efficacy of direct interventions to individuals.

There are three activities in which governments have an indispensable role in ensuring the efficiency and equity of prevention programs: providing public goods related to prevention, such as the collection and dissemination of information about the epidemic; reducing the negative externalities of risky behaviour by promoting safer behaviour among people who are most likely to contract and spread the virus; and promoting equity by ensuring that the most destitute are not denied access to the means by which they may protect themselves from HIV. These activities will reduce the spread of HIV most quickly and will benefit everyone in society, including those with low-risk behaviour and the poor. Private individuals would not invest in them in sufficient quantity to slow the epidemic.

In addition to satisfying these criteria of public economics, government-sponsored preventive activities should be cost-effective. We will review some important factors that influence the cost-effectiveness of government actions and propose a set of public priorities for preventing HIV according to the stage of the HIV/AIDS epidemic.

While governments, in collaboration with private actors, have implemented many worthwhile programs, some of which have had demonstrable impact, there is a need for renewed effort to implement the activities that are likely to be most cost-effective from the government perspective in preventing the epidemic. Perhaps the major impediment to more effective, efficient, and equitable prevention is a lack of political commitment, first, to collect and disseminate the data on HIV prevalence, risk behaviour, the effectiveness of programs, and their costs, and, second, to work constructively with those at highest risk of contracting and spreading HIV to prevent infection.

These are important issues that national governments, international donors, and non-governmental organizations need to act on urgently. A substantial body of economic research, much of it in developing countries, has shown that actual and perceived costs and benefits, some of which can be affected by government policies, significantly influence private decisions about marriage, childbearing, and contraceptive use.

It is therefore reasonable to assume that sexual behaviour that spreads HIV can also be influenced by public policy. Similarly, studies have shown that under the right conditions drug users change their injecting behaviour to reduce the likelihood of being infected with HIV. Four types of policies are likely to yield positive results with regard to the HIV epidemic: providing various types of information, reducing the costs of using condoms, reducing the costs of using sterile injecting equipment, and attempting to raise the costs of engaging in commercial sex and injecting drug use. Knowledge about the levels of HIV infection in the population—how HIV is transmitted, and how to avoid contracting it—can induce some people who engage in high-risk behaviour to adopt safer sexual and injecting practices or to refrain from casual or commercial sex and injecting drug use altogether. Moreover, there is considerable evidence that people engaged ill high-risk activities are more motivated to learn about HIV than others, since they are more likely to become infected and suffer the consequences.

Surveys conducted by the Global Programme on AIDS in 1989-90 found that respondents who had engaged in risky behaviour knew more about modes of transmission and the severity of AIDS than those who had never engaged in risky behaviour. Researchers have identified a number of interrelated factors that affect the way in which people use knowledge to assess the costs and benefits of risky behaviour and internalize them. These factors include the extent to which they understand how HIV infection would affect them personally, now risky they perceive their own behaviour to be and they have the skills necessary to negotiate safer behaviour with partners and to resist social pressures. Interventions that address these issues can result in substantially more behaviour change than knowledge alone. These interventions can take many forms, from public information campaigns using mass media to training and education programs conducted face-to-face.

Many knowledgeable people who have the skills to reduce their risk and have internalized the dangers will continue to engage in risky behaviour. Given the devastating personal cost of contracting HIV, why isn't the danger of being infected sufficient to cause people to forgo all risky activities? One reason is that the costs of reducing risk are clear and immediate while the benefits are uncertain and distant. Whether people are willing to incur these up-front costs to reduce the risk of future sickness and premature death from AIDS depends on their assessment of the probability of infection from a specific act and the discount rate applied to future years of healthy life. Assessing the probability of infection is not easy, since most people do not know the HIV infection, status of their partners or even the extent of their partners' current or past risky behaviour.

It is hardly surprising that, for people in the thrall of passion, addiction, or difficult economic circumstances, the immediate and certain costs of reducing their risk of contracting HIV will sometimes appear greater than the uncertain future benefits. Moreover, even if people making decisions about their private behaviour take into full account the potential costs to themselves, they are likely to greatly undervalue the costs of their behaviour to society in terms of secondary infections that unintentionally may result. For these reasons, although better information on the risks will induce people engaging in high-risk behaviour to reduce their somewhat, they will still engage in riskier behaviour than society would prefer in the interest of curbing the AIDS epidemic.

Additional measures will be necessary to change the costs and benefits of risky behaviour and its alternatives in ways that encourage safer behaviour. The costs of condom use include not only the price of the condom but also the potential inconvenience and embarrassment of obtaining and using one, and, for some people, reduced sexual pleasure. Policies that lower these costs, by lowering the price of condoms, improving their availability, and increasing their social acceptability, would be expected to increase condom use and reduce HIV transmission. Condom social marketing programs aim to achieve all of these objectives. These programs are often targeted at low-income households, where the price of condoms is more likely to inhibit demand. Following the introduction of condom social marketing programs, sales have increased dramatically.

In many of the countries condoms were virtually unavailable or unknown prior to the program. Most condom social marketing programs are subsidized by international donors and many, such as the program in India, receive government subsidies. Some governments have also lowered condom prices by reducing import tariffs and sales taxes on condoms and latex rubber. Some governments, NGOs, and condom social marketing programs also have launched for condom promotion focused specifically on commercial sex. Some of these programs distribute condoms to sex workers for free. Several NGOs have succeeded in raising condom use among sex workers and have shown decrease in cases. Policies to increase condom use among people who have unprotected sex with many partners are a potentially powerful means of reducing the size of the HIV epidemic and thereby of providing significant benefit to the entire society.

Since HIV greatly increases the personal cost of injecting with shared equipment, we would expect to see substantial behavioural change, provided there are low-cost ways for injecting drug users to avoid becoming infected. Not all injecting drug users are addicted, but for those who are, quitting is rarely a low-cost option. It can be extremely painful, can take a long time, and is often not successful: within a year or two of completing drug treatment, 70 to 80 per cent of people treated for heroin use typically resume injecting. Although treatment often does not result in permanent cessation of drug use, it can sometimes result in less risky behaviour, lower injecting rates and less needle sharing among those who resume injecting.

Thus, by providing information on the risks of HIV transmission and lowering the costs of drug treatment programs, it may induce some injecting drug users to stop injecting altogether and others to adopt safer practices. Many are likely to continue risky injecting behaviour unless the costs of safer injecting behaviour—primarily the costs of obtaining sterile equipment or bleach—are sufficiently low. But in many countries safer injecting behaviour can be very costly to the injecting drug user. Research suggests that difficulty in obtaining sterile injecting equipment is the most important reason that injecting drug users share equipment.

One inexpensive way for governments to lower the cost of safer injecting behaviour is to remove legal barriers to the purchase and possession of sterile injecting equipment. When armed with knowledge of the risks and provided with, easy access to sterile equipment, injecting drug users in many countries have rapidly adopted safer behaviour. Needle exchange programs, by providing new sterile injecting equipment in exchange for used syringes, minimize needle sharing and remove contaminated needles from circulation.

Many NEPs also supply free condoms to help prevent the spread of HIV to the sexual partners of injecting drug users, as well as education about reducing high-risk behaviour and referral for drug treatment. NEPs have been widely adopted in Australia, New Zealand, and many Western European countries with great success in reducing transmission of HIV as well as other blood-borne infections, like hepatitis B and hepatitis C. A recent study compared trends in HIV prevalence among injecting users in a sample of 81 cities in North America, Europe, and Asia and the South Pacific. In the 52 cities without NEPs, HIV prevalence among injecting drug users increased by 5.9 per cent per year, on average, while it declined by an almost equal per cent annually (5.8 percent) in the 29 cities that had NEPs.

A national NEP in the United States would have prevented from 4,000 to 10,000 HIV infections between 1987 and 1995 among drug users, their sexual partners, and children; if such a program had been implemented in 1996, it could still have prevented from 5,000 to 11,000 infections over the next five years. Can harm reduction strategies also work in low-income countries? The answer appears to be yes. Although there is less experience with harm reduction strategies in developing countries, the remarkable success of a needle exchange program in Nepal suggests that such programs should be attempted more widely. Where resources for needle exchange are lacking, bleach distribution may offer a less expensive alternative. Bleach is not only cheaper, it is also less controversial than needle exchanges, and, when used correctly, highly effective in killing HIV on infected equipment.

Furthermore, improved availability of bleach is virtually the only option for harm reduction among injecting drug users in prisons, since prison authorities are unlikely to distribute needles because they can be used as weapons. However, bleach is not always readily available. Bleach programs produce the greatest gains. Programs that reduce the cost of safer injecting procedures often arouse fears that they will encourage people to initiate drug use or discourage addicts from seeking treatment. If efforts to reduce the cost of safer injection behaviour did encourage illicit drug use, this would have to be weighed against the benefits of reduced HIV transmission. Fortunately, there is substantial evidence indicating that this is not the case.

Two evaluations of NEPs in six industrial countries failed to find any evidence that the programs raised the number of injecting drug users or that they increased the number of properly discarded needles. We have seen that lowering the costs of safer sex and safer injecting behaviour can encourage less-risky behaviour and reduce the transmission of HIV.

But both prostitution and use of illegal and addictive drugs impose substantial negative externalities on society in terms of sexually transmitted and blood-borne diseases, crime, the costs of law enforcement, and incarceration. It is not surprising, therefore, that programs that attempt to promote safer behaviour among sex workers, injecting drug users, and other people who engage in high-risk behaviour may be politically unpopular, especially if they are perceived to be condoning prostitution or drug addiction.

An alternative approach that often has broad popular appeal is to discourage such activities through punitive measures and stepped up enforcement of existing laws. From the standpoint of economic theory, such attempts to raise the cost of potentially risky behaviour could discourage it, provided that costs can be raised sufficiently. However, because sexual activity and injecting drug use are private activities, enforcing prohibitions is costly and difficult in practice. Such attempts may have unintended consequences that may exacerbate the epidemic.

Numerous studies have shown that prohibition and punishment of commercial sex causes sex workers to shift their place of business and to change the way they solicit clients to avoid prosecution. Singapore, for example, attempted to eradicate prostitution by closing "red-light" districts in commercial areas; brothels soon appeared in residential areas. Enforcement problems aside, punishing commercial sex is also not very efficient in preventing HIV, because the virus is transmitted not by commercial sex per se but by unprotected intercourse with multiple partners, regardless of whether one party pays the other.

Thus, even if commercial sex could be eliminated by these measures, HIV could persist and spread through casual sex networks, although perhaps less rapidly. Moreover, it is reasonable to expect that the more effective is the curtailment of commercial sex, the more casual sex networks will expand. An alternative to prohibiting and punishing commercial sex is to legalize and regulate it.

Although this approach sometimes arouses considerable political opposition, it can make sex workers and their clients easier to monitor and to reach with information, condoms, and STD treatment. The likely result is a legal, high-priced market, presumably with lower transmission of HIV, and an unregulated, low-priced Market, which authorities cannot easily monitor and where transmission of HIV will presumably be higher. Moreover, mandatory health screening of prostitutes, even in the regulated brothels, is not always enforceable.

The net impact of legalization and regulation is also difficult to predict and will depend on how much regulation raises the price of sex in the legalized sector and the extent to which programs are successful in encouraging safer sex in the illegal, unregulated sector. Arguments for and against raising the costs of drug use through prohibition and punishment are broadly similar to those for prohibiting commercial sex. Again, it is important to note that neither drug use per se nor injecting per se spreads HIV; rather, it is the sharing of unsterilized equipment that does so. Many who use illicit drugs do not inject, and often those who inject do not share needles. So efforts to eliminate illegal drug use, while they might be rationalized on other grounds, are potentially a very inefficient and costly way of reducing the unsafe injecting behaviour that spreads HIV.

The already substantial political appeal of drug enforcement efforts is likely to be strengthened by the close association between use of injected drugs and HIV. It is therefore useful to consider the likely impact on HIV of the two main strategies for eradicating illegal drugs: restricting supply, by attempting to halt the drug trade, and reducing demand, by punishing drug users or forcing them into treatment. The most politically popular way to attempt to reduce drug use is to reduce the availability of drugs. However, drug interdiction may simply rearrange the problem or make it worse. For example:

— Addicts may switch to other substances.

— May shift from smoking to injecting, which requires a smaller dose to produce euphoria but greatly raises the risk of HIV.

— The drug trade may shift to other areas where people not previously exposed to drugs may begin injecting.

Because most injecting drug users are chemically dependent, prohibition and threats of punishment are notoriously ineffective in reducing their demand for drugs. A survey of 450 injecting drug users in Manipur State in India, where addicts are imprisoned, found that only 2 per cent regarded the threat of imprisonment as a reason to stop injecting drugs; half of the addicts surveyed had previously been in prison.

Far from reducing HIV transmission, imprisonment may have the opposite effect. Unable to obtain syringes, prisoners who inject drugs frequently resort to shared, improvised equipment, such as ballpoint pens, which would be very difficult to sterilize, even if bleach were available. Mandatory drug treatment is likely to be even less successful in ending drug use than voluntary treatment, since patients entering such programs presumably have very little desire to change their behaviour. Efforts to raise the cost of injecting drugs through drug interdiction or the punishment of injecting drug users may increase rather than decrease risky injection behaviour.

Although the data on the impact of such efforts on HIV incidence are fragmentary, the available evidence suggests that harm reduction programs, including information about HIV, sterile injection equipment or bleach kits, and referral for voluntary treatment programs will be more effective and less costly in reducing risky injection behaviour than drug interdiction or incarceration of addicts.

A second approach to reducing the spread of HIV aims to change the social and economic factors that shape—and sometimes constrain—individual choices about risky behaviour. Measures pursued by this approach have many other benefits besides reducing the HIV epidemic and they are already on the agenda of most developing country governments. The benefits are sometimes more difficult to quantify because of their broad impact, which extends far beyond HIV prevention. However, these measures are highly complementary to policies that directly affect the costs and benefits of risky behaviour. Social norms and peer pressure that encourage men to use the services of prostitutes or that venerate men with many female "conquests," while placing a high value on female chastity create the conditions for an explosive HIV epidemic.

The challenge for policymakers in countries with social patterns that are very conducive to the spread of HIV is to encourage safer behaviour, without stigmatizing those who engage in unsafe behaviour in ways that make them more difficult to reach with public health interventions. Norms on marriage and childbearing can also affect the spread and prevention of HIV.

The tradition of a man selecting a bride who is five or ten years younger than himself spreads HIV from one generation to the next. Finally, efforts to encourage condom use among married couples for HIV prevention will be especially difficult in societies where people want large families and a woman's social status and economic well-being are heavily dependent on the number of children she has. While sexual conservatism may be one of the best protections against HIV at the societal level, adherence to norms is never complete.

An HIV epidemic can nevertheless occur, and conservatism can result in stigma of those who become infected or who are in social groups associated with high-risk behaviour, making it more difficult to support safer behaviour. The lower social and economic status of women reduces their ability to insist upon male sexual fidelity and to negotiate safe sex. These problems can be particularly acute in societies where women's inheritance rights, property and child custody, rights in divorce, and even the right to own land and other property are limited. In some instances, a wife's mere suggestion that her husband use a condom can provoke physical abuse. Even where the situation is not this stark, women's lower literacy, lower incomes, and low economic independence give them less access to HIV prevention information, fewer resources to purchase condoms and treat conventional STDs, and less ability to leave a relationship that puts them at risk of contracting HIV.

For all these reasons, many more women than men face situations in which they are unable to protect them from HIV. Women who sell sexual services often face particularly constrained choices. Unemployment, divorce, desertion, and the breakdown of the extended family are among the factors that can lead women to offer sex for money. One-half of sex workers interviewed in Calcutta cited extreme poverty as the reason for entering sex work, and 22 per cent cited "family disturbances". Ending legal restrictions on women's rights, encouraging social equality, and raising economic opportunities for women not only make it easier for women to avoid HIV, they are also important in fostering development.

Policies that specifically help women include increasing girls' school enrolment; guaranteeing equal employment opportunities; outlawing and severely punishing slavery, rape, wife abuse, and child prostitution; and guaranteeing inheritance, property, and child custody rights. A growing economy is also an important ingredient for increased economic opportunities for women.

Of course, improving the status of women will also open new opportunities to choose risky behaviour; a few women may do so. However, it is reasonable to expect that the vast majority of women, given expanded choices, would seize the opportunity to choose safe behaviour and avoid HIV infection. Poverty and low socio-economic status also constrain the decisions people make about risky behaviour. Those with low incomes, for example, may not be able to afford to treat STDs or to buy condoms.

Poor families may see commercial sex as a lucrative occupation for young and poorly educated daughters. People with less education may have less access to information about the dangers of high-risk behaviour or be less able to understand prevention messages. This explains why those most likely to contract STDs and other infectious diseases within a society are the poor and uneducated. However, studies have proved that people with higher socio-economic status have higher HIV infection rates.

The first reason is that men with higher education and income will find it easier to attract and support additional commercial and casual sexual partners. Analysis of data from the WHO/GPA sexual behaviour surveys found that in five African sites, as well as in Thailand, Manila (the Philippines), and Rio de Janeiro (Brazil), the more education a man has, the more likely he is to have had a casual, nonregular sexual partner.

A second reason is that men and women with more education and higher incomes are likely to travel more and thus have more opportunities for a variety of sexual contacts. Several studies of sex workers have found that women with higher incomes were more likely to use condoms and had lower levels of HIV infection.

In three cities in Sao Paulo, Brazil, for example, sex workers who charged higher prices had fewer clients, were more likely to have always used condoms in the past year, were less likely to have injected drugs, and consequently were less likely to be infected with HIV and other STDs than were low-priced sex workers. Despite the links found between higher socioeconomic status and HIV infection in some areas, government policies to raise incomes and schooling and reduce poverty should lower the economic constraints to engaging in safer behaviour and reduce the incidence of HIV over the long term.

These policies are often pursued because they have far-reaching social benefits; they are also highly complementary to short-term interventions to encourage safer sexual and injecting behaviour and will likely enhance the impact of these interventions. This section proposes a broad prevention strategy for governments at all stages of the epidemic to maximize the impact of limited government resources in curbing the spread of HIV.

In keeping with the principles of public economics, governments should finance or directly implement interventions that are essential to stopping the spread of HIV because private individuals or firms will not have sufficient incentive to finance on their own—namely, provision of public goods, reduction of the negative externalities of behaviour that spreads HIV, and protection of the poor from HIV infection.

Programs that address these issues will improve the efficiency and equity of government prevention efforts.

Program effectiveness will be improved if governments act as soon as possible and if they succeed in preventing infection among those most likely to contract and spread HIV.

The intention is to identify the minimum set of activities that all governments should be engaged in to improve the efficiency and equity of prevention programs, and a rational order in which to expand them. This strategy should be broad one, based on underlying principles of public economics, epidemiology, and cost-effectiveness. It remains for individual countries to identify the specific combination of programs, policies, and interventions to pursue this strategy in a cost-effective way.

However, even within these guiding principles, the cost-effectiveness of HIV prevention programs is likely to vary considerably according to the setting. Programmatic choices are necessarily country-specific because the costs and effectiveness of interventions, as well as the characteristics and accessibility of those most likely to contract and spread HIV, vary widely across the globe. Government policies can potentially address three types of market failures that occur with respect to the prevention of HIV.

The first problem involves the underprovision of public good-specifically, the lack of incentives for the private sector to collect and disseminate information crucial to the prevention of the epidemic.

The second involves the negative externalities of high-risk behaviour: people deciding whether or not to take steps to protect themselves from HIV are likely to consider the costs to themselves of becoming infected but may not consider the cost of secondary HIV infections that may result if they become infected.

The third type of market failure involves equity: very poor people are less able to protect themselves against HIV than others.

The collection and production of information about the prevention and control of HIV is almost entirely a public good. Essential information includes data on the levels and trends of HIV and STD infections, the prevalence of high-risk behaviour, and the costs and benefits of prevention programs.

Unprotected intercourse with multiple partners and unsafe injecting practices raise the risk of infection for everyone, even for those who do not engage in high-risk behaviour. People who practice risky behaviour are likely to take some steps to reduce their risk of contracting HIV because of the enormous personal costs if they become infected.

However, because they react primarily to the increased risk to themselves, their response will not reflect the full costs—that is, the negative externalities—of unintentionally spreading HIV to the rest of society. Many people who do not practice high-risk behaviour would be willing to pay those who do practice it to adopt safer behaviour in order to contain the epidemic and thus lower everyone's risk of contracting HIV.

Government is the only mechanism through which this can happen. Thus, there is a strong justification for government to subsidize safer behaviour among people who engage in high-risk behaviour in order to protect everyone—either by preventing primary infections among those who engage in high-risk behaviour or, when such individuals are already infected, by preventing the infection from spreading to others.

The principles of public economics and epidemiology are therefore in agreement that governments should give high priority to the prevention of infection among people most likely to contract and spread HIV. The extent of negative externalities of risky behaviour can be measured by the number of secondary infections that a person would generate if infected with HIV. By this definition, the riskier an individual's behaviour, the more secondary infections he or she is likely to generate, and thus the greater the negative externalities of his or her behaviour. The reproductive rate of HIV among such individuals is likely to be much greater than 1, sustaining the epidemic. They are vulnerable to the negative externalities generated by others' risky behaviour. In countries where government has a broad mandate to provide health services to everyone, and where resources are adequate, expanding government-financed preventive interventions to the low-risk population should not be ruled out.

However, even in these cases, governments should first ensure that programs achieve adequate coverage of those most likely to contract and spread HIV, starting from those with the highest-risk behaviour, since this is the most efficient way to protect everyone. There are situations, however, in which interventions for the entire population are essential to the success of programs aimed at reaching those most likely to contract and spread HIV. For example, although information that helps people with low-risk behaviour to further reduce their risk will have very little impact on the overall epidemic, they need to understand how HIV is transmitted and—more important—how it is not transmitted.

Inaccurate information or even accurate information presented in ways that create feelings of fear and vulnerability can incite discrimination against those who are at high risk of contracting and spreading HIV and people who are HIV-positive or living with AIDS. This is not only unwarranted and unjust, but it may also compromise the ability to launch the prevention programs most likely to slow the spread of HIV. Information that fuels fear of HIV-infected people has been a serious problem in nearly all countries where there has been extensive early publicity about the epidemic.

Government's first step should be to lower the costs of safe behaviour for the poor by improving the functioning of markets, for example, by eliminating tariffs on condoms and restrictions on condom advertising. If prevention is still too costly for the poor, subsidies may also be warranted. In countries where particular groups face significant barriers to acquiring information because of illiteracy, different languages, or lack of access to newspapers, radio or television-subsidized information for the disadvantaged groups will not improve their access to prevention.

Besides subsidized information about HIV, the most important preventive measures are those that make it easier for poor people to obtain condoms, treatment for STDs, and access to safe blood. However, unless there is substantial overlap between the poor and those with high-risk behaviour, subsidized HIV interventions for the poor will address equity but will not be sufficient to contain the epidemic, particularly in its early stages.

Cost-effectiveness analysis is a tool for deciding among alternative courses of action when resources are scarce. It seeks to determine how to achieve the maximum effect within a given budget or, viewed differently how to achieve a desired effect at the lowest possible cost. Measures for which individuals would have paid on their own are not a priority for a government's limited funds. Rather, governments should first spend their limited resources on interventions that are cost-effective in the conventional sense and that would not occur in the absence of government involvement—that is, cost-effective interventions that provide public goods and reduce the negative externalities of high-risk behaviour.

This strategy will ultimately prevent the largest number of subsequent infections among all subgroups in the population, including the majority who do not engage in high-risk behaviour. Some governments have the mandate to intervene broadly in the health sector and to assume responsibility for providing curative and preventive health care for all citizens, irrespective of whether government spending is efficiency enhancing.

However unless the costs of changing behaviour among those most likely to contract and spread HIV are extraordinarily high, promoting behaviour change among them is likely to be the most cost-effective in terms of preventing infection in the general population. Several factors that affect the cost-effectiveness of alternative, publicly financed by HIV/AIDS prevention programs, do not necessarily enter into cost-effectiveness calculations for private individuals. There are also a number of issues specific to the cost-effectiveness of HIV interventions that need to be taken into account.

In calculating the benefits from prevention programs, it is important to consider not only the benefits received by the person directly affected, but also the number of secondary infections that are averted. Secondary infections measure, in effect, the extent to which negative externalities are being addressed by programs. Failure to include secondary infections among the benefits of public health programs will result in serious underestimates of the benefits of prevention in groups that are very likely to contract and spread HIV. Even the number of people in these groups tends to be small so far as the total population is concerned, the number of secondary infections per person tends to be large.

Public programs will be more cost-effective if they raise additional demand for risk-reducing behaviour without "crowding out" private sources of inputs. For example, in societies where condoms are already widely available at low cost, subsidized condom projects that are not specifically directed toward those most likely to contract and spread HIV may simply shift the financing of existing condom sales from private pockets to public ones, with no impact on the epidemic. Whether the resulting redistribution enhances equity depends on the income distribution of condom purchasers relative to the general population. The effectiveness of public programs should therefore be measured as the difference between outcomes with and without the program. HIV/AIDS prevention has other external effects: many HIV/AIDS preventive interventions have additional positive effects that might be overlooked if cost-effectiveness calculations considered only the impact on HIV/AIDS.

Condom programs also prevent other STDs, which are spread in the same ways as HIV and generate similar negative externalities. HIV education in the schools and encouragement of condom use among adolescents who engage in sex will complement efforts to postpone sexual activity, reduce teenage pregnancy and abortion, and as a result improve school completion rate, among girls.

Harm reduction programs among injecting drug user, generate demand for drug rehabilitation programs and reduce transmission of hepatitis B and C and other blood-borne diseases. Although these benefits are difficult to quantify, they should not be overlooked. Involving other factors can improve cost-effectiveness: while governments must support prevention efforts among those who are most likely to contract and spread HIV, governments are not necessarily the most effective agent to design and implement such programs. Enlisting and subsidizing NGOs to help in the design and implementation of interventions can greatly improve the cost-effectiveness of public programs, particularly if the NGOs are staffed by or representative of people at high risk of contracting and spreading HIV.

The cost-effectiveness of all interventions can also be improved through other government measures, such as relaxing legal prohibitions and minimizing the stigma that people in high-risk subpopulations often face, so that NGOs can work more effectively. In the baseline scenario, before any intervention, we assume that only 20 per cent of sex workers and 5 per cent of men having sex with casual or commercial partners use condoms consistently, that is, in every act of intercourse. We also assume that none of the women in steady relationships are using condoms. The simulations show the impact of instantaneously raising consistent condom use among sex workers to 90 percent, and among the other two groups to 20 percent. These levels were selected because the authors believed that they are realistically achievable in some countries.

In other countries, it may be possible to exceed the levels of condom use simulated here. Among those who use condoms, the failure rate through breakage or misuse is assumed to be 5 percent. The simulations also show the impact of increased STD treatment on HIV prevalence. The baseline scenario assumes that 25 per cent of all STD cases that produce symptoms are effectively treated and that there is no specific screening or treatment program for sex workers. The simulations show the impact of increasing the share of symptomatic STDs treated to 75 per cent in the general population and, in a separate scenario, the impact of implementing a monthly screening and treatment program that covers 90 per cent of sex workers. In the latter intervention, it is assumed that 5 per cent of sex workers are not cured. Despite the different underlying patterns of sexual behaviour, the impact of specific interventions shows some striking consistencies across populations:

— Achieving 90 per cent condom use among sex workers results in a dramatic drop in HIV prevalence in all three populations where there is commercial sex, even though sex workers comprise only a very small share of each population (0.25 per cent or fewer women). STD screening and treatment for sex workers is far less powerful.

— Increased STD treatment among the general population is less effective than raising condom use among those with many partners. This is not surprising, since people with high-risk behaviour generate a disproportionate number of STD cases, and condoms prevent transmission of both HIV and STDs. STD treatment among the general population and condom use by women in stable relationships have the largest impact in the populations with concurrent casual sex.

— The impact of greater condom use among women in stable relationships is very small, and in the serial monogamy population it has almost no impact on the epidemic. In the population where the epidemic is driven by commercial sex, condom use by Monogamous women slightly accelerates a decline in HIV prevalence, while in the other two populations it merely slows the growth of a still-expanding epidemic.

— In the epidemic fuelled by commercial sex alone, all of the interventions produce an absolute decline in HIV prevalence; in the epidemic fuelled solely by casual sex, none of the simulated interventions is sufficient to cause an absolute decline.

— In the population with concurrent commercial and casual sex, prevalence declines in response to 90 per cent condom use among sex workers; 20 per cent condom use by men in casual sex keeps prevalence from rising. Other interventions in this population merely slow the expanding epidemic.

— In the population practising serial monogamy, increased condom use by sex workers is the only intervention that results in an absolute decline in HIV prevalence.

There is always spillover between interventions intended for people with different rates of partner change, so any particular intervention is likely to change behaviour in more than one group of people but to differing degrees. Further, combined interventions to multiple groups will have greater impact than single interventions; for example, working only with sex workers to raise condom use will be less effective than simultaneously working with both sex workers and their clients.

However, these simulations show that greatest share of the impact will be achieved through the interventions that succeed in changing the behaviour of those with the highest rates of partner change. Although the overall pattern of sexual behaviour in the population does affect the impact of interventions, prevention of infection among those with the highest rates of partner change has a large effect irrespective of the underlying patterns of sexual behaviour in the population. Assuming that it is not a great deal more expensive to increase rates of condom use among those with high rates of partner change—sex workers or other—focusing condom subsidies and promotion efforts on changing their behaviour is likely to be highly cost-effective. Studies of the cost-effectiveness of HIV interventions in developing countries are rare and not transferable. Fewer than half a dozen studies have documented the costs and effects of preventive interventions in developing countries.

Most evaluation studies measure impact by changes in intermediate behaviours that are believed to affect risk-such as the increase in condom use, or knowledge about HIV prevention, or the number of people receiving sterile syringes. The number of HIV infections averted is then extrapolated on the basis of assumptions about the relationship between the behaviour and HIV incidence. However, the lack of good data on sexual behaviour and on the relation between sexual behaviour and incidence makes these benefits very difficult to assess.

Virtually no studies, except those based on simulations, have measured the impact of interventions on secondary cases where they are thought to exist. None to our knowledge have taken into account the external benefits of interventions or the issue of complementarities between interventions. While cost-effectiveness studies can be very useful in deciding among alternative interventions in a given setting and stage of the epidemic, their conclusions are usually not easily transferable to other settings. Ideally, we would like to know the costs and effects of alternative interventions implemented in the same setting, but this has rarely been done. Interventions focused on those most likely to contract and spread HIV should be more cost-effective from the public perspective, because preventing infection in a person with risky behaviour prevents many secondary infections among individuals with whom they mix—some of whom practice high-risk behaviour and some of whom practice lower-risk behaviour. In fact, the extent to which ongoing programs affect those who practice high-risk behaviour is often unknown.

Although it is highly desirable to focus public interventions on those who are most likely to contract and spread HIV, identifying and reaching these individuals can be difficult, especially where legal sanctions and social stigma cause these people to want to avoid being discovered. The costs of reaching those most likely to contract and spread the virus can have a significant impact on the cost-effectiveness of intervention. Since individuals with high-risk behaviour cannot be easily identified, programs need to focus interventions on people with characteristics that are highly correlated with risky behaviour.

However, some sex workers consistently use condoms, and some government employees who have many partners do not. Intervening to change the behaviour of people with specific characteristics like age, sex, occupation, or geographic area is not a perfect way to reach those with high-risk behaviour. The lack of perfect criteria for focusing interventions on those with the highest-risk behaviours is one source of leakage of program resources. This reduces the cost-effectiveness of interventions if resources go to people with lower-risk behaviour. On the other hand, leakage may improve cost- effectiveness if resources go to people with even riskier behaviour than those targeted.

Surveys of sexual behaviour, such as those conducted by WHO/GPA and DHS, can help to overcome these problems by establishing the characteristics and geographic location of those who have unprotected sex and high rates of partner change. Unless programs are carefully designed and implemented, targeting prevention programs to groups with specific characteristics may stigmatize members and lead to discrimination, making future prevention efforts more difficult and less effective. There must be a broad prevention strategy that assigns priority to activities based on the principles of epidemiology, public economics, and cost-effectiveness. Whatever the stage of the epidemic, this strategy calls for a strong emphasis on prevention activities starting with those at highest risk of contracting and spreading HIV and covering as many others as available resources allow.

As the epidemic expands, it will increasingly require efforts to prevent infection among people with relatively lower levels of risk, which will raise the cost of prevention activities. If the epidemic is to be contained, this expansion of activities must not weaken the fundamental commitment to work with those most likely to contract and spread the virus. Provision of public goods or ensuring their provision by regulation is an important role for government at all stages of an HIV/AIDS epidemic. Governments should invest in the information-collecting infrastructure they need to monitor the epidemic and to identify where high-risk behaviours are practised and how to reach those at highest risk.

In a nascent epidemic, understanding levels of HIV and STD infection in the subpopulations most likely to contract and spread HIV, the underlying patterns of sexual behaviour, and the nature of the links to lower-risk subpopulations are critical pieces of information for assessing the probability of a more extensive epidemic. As the epidemic progresses, governments need to monitor, in addition, the spread of HIV to populations at lower risk and to support evaluation of the costs and effectiveness of alternative interventions.

The need to reduce the negative externalities of high-risk behaviour, as well as the insights of epidemiology, argue for heavily subsidizing safer behaviour among those most likely to contract and spread HIV in countries at all stages of the HIV/AIDS epidemic.

It is not necessary to wait for HIV to take hold to make widespread knowledge, 100 per cent condom use, and quick recognition and treatment of other STDs the norm among those more likely to contract and spread HIV, such as sex workers, bar maids, long-distance truck drivers, the military and police, millers or factory workers living away from home, and homosexual and bisexual men with multiple partners. The case for rapid action is even stronger in the case of injecting drug users because of the potential for very rapid increases in HIV prevalence in this subpopulation, and the subsequent spread of HIV to others, including their sex partners (some of whom may be sex workers) and their children.

In a nascent HIV epidemic, such highly focused actions may be sufficient to dramatically slow the spread of the virus. In countries with concentrated and generalized epidemics, preventing HIV among those with the highest chances of contracting and spreading the virus is still essential to slowing the epidemic.

However, behaviour change among with less-risky behaviour who may nonetheless inadvertently spread the virus will be necessary to reverse the course of the epidemic. With respect to ensuring equity, in countries with nascent epidemics, government can protect the poor best by acting early and decisively to prevent an epidemic. In countries with generalized epidemics, the risk of infection has risen for everyone and poverty should not restrict access to preventive services.

Government can ensure that the poor have access to the knowledge, skills, and means to prevent HIV. The cost-effectiveness of interventions aimed at people with different levels of risky behaviour will also change as HIV spreads from those who practice more risky behaviour to those at relatively lower risk. Interventions for those most likely to contract and spread HIV are still likely to be highly cost-effective. In countries where HIV has spread widely in the general population, the cost-effectiveness of preventive interventions for lower-risk populations, such as subsidies for STD treatment, provision of safe blood, and reproductive health and AIDS education in schools, improves.

However, these programs do not generate many externalities: their benefits accrue mainly to the person who uses them. While such interventions will prevent HIV infections and save lives, they will not do so as efficiently as interventions focused on those more likely to contract and spread HIV and they will often not be sufficient to reverse the course of the epidemic. Furthermore, the costs of providing these services to the entire population at low risk of spreading HIV are potentially very large. In light of the substantial individual benefits of these services, people who are not poor will usually be willing and able to pay for them.

In countries with scarce financial resources, the priority should be first on guaranteeing equity in access to these services by the poor. Not all developing countries face equal resource constraints in pursuing this strategy. In the lowest- income countries, prevention should start among those whose behaviour generates or is likely to generate the higher reproductive rate for HIV; subsidized prevention to others with lower HIV reproductive rates that are still greater than 1 can be extended as resources permit.

Middle-income countries may have the resources, even in the earliest stages of the epidemic, to finance interventions for a much larger share of those for whom the HIV reproductive rates would be greater than 1. They may also have the resources to subsidize to a greater extent services for the poor and to extend prevention subsidies to sub-populations that are unlikely to spread HIV to others. At an operational level it is impossible to determine the actual or potential reproductive rate of HIV for any group of individuals. However, using information about the average number of partners, condom use, and injecting behaviour from surveys and epidemiological surveillance, subpopulations in a given country can be ranked from those with the highest-risk behaviour those most likely to contract and spread HIV to those with the lowest-risk behaviour.

Once the highest-priority subpopulations have been effectively reached, programs can be expanded to cover those with progressively less-risky behaviour, provided that sufficient resources are available. Indeed, if sustained behaviour change is achieved in the highest-priority groups, the relative priority assigned to other groups will increase. Of course, no ranking of this sort can apply to all countries, or even to a single country over time. To overcome problems in locating the people most likely to contract and spread HIV at any given point in time, it is essential that policymakers and program managers finance collection of the necessary information for cost-effective use of the scarce resources available for HIV prevention. Countries at the nascent stage of the epidemic have a unique opportunity to act early, to make a few key investments, and largely prevent an HIV epidemic. Not all countries with low levels of infection will necessarily go on to experience an HIV epidemic, even without government action.

However, our inadequate understanding of the distribution of different behaviours in the population and the links between different subpopulations make it difficult to predict which among the countries will be so lucky and which will not. Furthermore, even in countries where high-risk behaviour is relatively rare, patterns of sexual and injecting behaviour can change with economic and social conditions. Interventions at the nascent stage are the most effective and will likely involve far less total cost than if implemented after HIV has saturated subpopulations with high-risk behaviour. These recommendations are not meant to limit the scope of government involvement if there are ample resources and public will to undertake even more. Rather, our intention is to point out the minimum set of activities that all governments should be engaged in to improve the efficiency and equity of prevention programs and a rational order in which to expand these activities if HIV spreads or more resources become available. The overwhelming impression left by the AIDS in the world-wide survey and national AIDS control plans started by many countries, is that many countries have launched a collection of AIDS prevention activities without clear-cut priorities; indeed, many programs do not focus on preventing infections among people most likely to contract and spread the virus. The lack of understanding the importance of spreading virus, domestic political considerations and the preferences of international donors for particular programs are probably also responsible.

Nevertheless, in such an environment, limited resources are likely to be stretched very thin, and the cost-effectiveness of public expenditure on prevention is likely to be low. The limited evidence available suggests that as much as one-quarter of all developing countries have yet to initiate systematic monitoring of HIV prevalence. A background study for

AIDS in the world-wide classified countries into four groups according to whether HIV sentinel surveillance sites were planned (but not yet operating), limited, many, or extensive. The good news is that countries at the generalized stage of the epidemic were most likely to have many or extensive sites, while those at the concentrated and nascent stages were most likely to have limited sites.

However, one in five developing countries at the nascent stage of the epidemic reported no sentinel surveillance sites, and for another 14 per cent the extent of sentinel surveillance was unknown. If we add all the countries reporting only planned sites to those countries for which information about sites was inadequate to determine their extent, we find that 27 countries—more than one-fifth of countries at all stages of the epidemic—were not reporting any operating HIV sentinel surveillance sites in January 1995. Even in those countries that have some form of sentinel surveillance, information on HIV prevalence among those most likely to contract and spread the virus is often lacking. Although delays in the receipt of reports probably account for some missing data, available information was insufficient to classify 31 developing countries by stage of the epidemic, usually because of a lack of information on those presumed on average to practice riskier behaviour—sex workers, injecting drug users, men who have sex with men, the military, and STD patients.

Among the 123 developing countries attempted to classify, 43 countries (35 per cent) had no information on HIV prevalence in any group with presumed high-risk behaviour during the last 5 years. While it is more convenient to monitor HIV trends among blood donors and women attending antenatal clinics, regular monitoring of HIV Prevalence early in the epidemic among those who practice high-risk behaviour is much more important. In addition to ensuring more and better monitoring of HIV prevalence, governments urgently need information on patterns of sexual behaviour, condom use, and drug-injecting behaviour. The heterogeneity of behaviour and the extent of mixing between people with high and low-risk behaviour determine the baseline shape of the AIDS epidemic.

Countries at all stages of the epidemic need information on the prevalence and distribution of risky behaviours among representative samples of men and women to understand the likely path of the epidemic and how the epidemic can be minimized. However, this information remains scarce. Fewer than 20 developing countries are known to have undertaken sexual behaviour surveys, such as those sponsored by GPA or DHS, that could provide such information. Evaluations of HIV prevention programs often fail to measure the costs of interventions or their impact, reporting instead on indicators of process and implementation. Information on costs and impact is important not only for assessing the most efficient allocation of resources, but also for demonstrating the effectiveness of interventions to change behaviour among those most likely to contract and spread HIV and the spillover benefits to the low-risk population.

Developing countries need better information on the costs and effects of pilot interventions, which interventions affect whose behaviour, and at what cost. Most countries have a few interventions that focus on people most likely to contract and spread HIV, but most of these programs achieve only limited coverage. To arrest the epidemic, the coverage of preventive measures directed toward these groups needs to be expanded considerably. Although many people practising high-risk behaviour are difficult to reach for prevention, some people whose circumstances may put them at higher risk of HIV infection are part of "captive" populations that can be readily identified: the military, police, and prisoners.

Because governments usually have much easier access to these organized groups than to injecting drug users, sex workers, or others with many casual partners. It should be possible for governments to reach nearly all members of each of these groups with preventive interventions only. The Civil-Military Alliance to combat HIV and AIDS conducted a survey of prevention activities among the militaries of 50 countries, about half of which were low and middle-income countries. Although individual country results are not available (countries were assured that responses would be confidential), the aggregate data clearly reveal that prevention programs in the military often fall short of complete coverage. Low coverage of other groups of people presumed to practice riskier-than-average behaviour can be seen in a small survey of UNAIDS Country Programme Advisers conducted for this report.

The survey asked the advisers who work in 32 developing countries to identify groups of people with high-risk behaviour and to comment on the extent to which programs focused on prevention in these groups; the approximate percentage of each group covered; and the extent of government encouragement and finance of these programs. Although the results reflect the assessment of the advisers rather than the national AIDS program managers and cannot be generalized beyond the countries surveyed, they nonetheless reveal tremendous scope for improving outreach to those who are most likely to contract and spread HIV. Respondents named adolescents as the subpopulation most likely to be the recipient of an intervention, financed either by government or the private sector. All countries had at least one program focused on youth, even though in many of the countries it is not clear to what extent adolescents engage in risky behaviour.

About nine out of ten countries reported a public or private program focused on sex workers, while about seven out of ten countries had a program focused on injecting drug users; a slightly lower proportion of countries had programs that focus on the military and on men who have sex with men. Respondents estimated that these programs on average covered only about one-half of the relevant group with high-risk behaviour. Coverage was highest for adolescents and the military, and lowest for men who have sex with men and injecting drug users. The UNAIDS Country Programme Advisers also reported that governments were least likely to finance and most likely to impede prevention programs targeted to men who have sex with men and injecting drug users. Although six out of ten governments funded prevention programs for adolescents, only about one-third did so for the military and for sex workers.

Two advisers indicated that the government in their country promoted prevention for the general population of heterosexuals, but neither encouraged nor discouraged programs for those most likely to contract and spread the virus. While some prevention programs have attempted to encourage safer behaviour among those most likely to contract and spread HIV, coverage is generally low. The fact that governments may have logistic and political difficulties in reaching groups such as sex workers and injecting drug users, while understandable, does not detract from the urgent need to assure the fullest possible coverage of these groups.

Often these obstacles can be overcome through government funding and support of NGOs. Moreover, in many countries coverage is low even among "captive" populations, such as the military; where this is the case, governments have an opportunity to inexpensively reach these groups with information and other prevention interventions. Effective interventions with broad coverage of those with high-risk behaviour will go a long way toward preventing infection among others engaging in high-risk activities and among the lower-risk population. The effectiveness of government programs in ensuring access to prevention for the poor has rarely been evaluated. However, improving equity of access to condoms is one of the major objectives of condom social marketing programs and free government distribution of condoms.

Condom availability and use in general have expanded considerably, partly as a spontaneous response to HIV and partly as a result of social marketing and other public, private, and donor-sponsored programmes. As of 1996, 60 developing countries had functioning condom social marketing programs, although not all were on a national scale. The extent to which these programs disproportionately help poor people to obtain condoms is not clear.

In most countries, people with higher incomes and education are more likely to use condoms. Providing subsidized condoms to low-risk individuals who would have purchased them at market prices, would neither improve equity nor reduce the epidemic. Likewise, while condom use has risen in both the subsidized and commercial market, it is still not clear the extent to which subsidized programmes have squeezed out private sales. This is likely to be an important issue in older condom social marketing programmes, after their initial effect on popularizing condoms and generating greater demand has worn off.

Another way in which these programs promote equity is by encouraging condom use among those most likely to contract and spread HIV, forestalling or slowing the epidemic before it reaches the poor. Unfortunately, relatively little is known about the extent to which condom social marketing programs are used by those with the highest rates of partner change—which is the key to their effectiveness in slowing the epidemic. Surveys of sexually active adults confirm that people are far more likely to use a condom for sex with a casual or extramarital partner than a steady partner or a spouse. But they do not show whether these programmes reach people with the highest rates of partner change. Do these programs lower the costs of condom use sufficiently to bring about high-use rates among sex workers, soldiers, truck drivers, and other people with many partners? By selling through nontraditional outlets like bars and hotels, condom social marketing programs are probably much more likely to reach people with risky behaviour than are conventional programs that distribute condoms through health clinics. The condom program may also fail to reach those with the highest rates of partner change. For example, sex workers and young, sexually active men do not frequent by visit health or family planning clinics.

Furthermore, women who need condoms for STD prevention may be reluctant to obtain them from community health or family planning clinics, even if free of charge, because of inconvenience, an unreliable supply, or a desire for anonymity. These problems can be overcome if condoms are promoted specifically for HIV and STD prevention and if they can be readily and cheaply obtained in nontraditional outlets readily accessible to people in situations that tend to be conducive to casual and commercial sex. One way for governments to stimulate demand for condoms for disease prevention is to end restrictions on condom advertising. But even when there are no legal barriers, open promotion of condom use can be extremely controversial if it is seen as encouraging promiscuity.

Messages must convey useful information and at the same time be directed to the appropriate populations so as to avoid offending influential leaders and segments of the public. When a virus encounters a new host, it will remain if it can establish itself rapidly enough for transmission. Even if adaptation is long and difficult, the virus will remain as long as it can maintain at least some level of spread in the new population. If the host environment accommodates the newcomer well enough, an optimal equilibrium can be found between virus survival and host survival. This equilibrium may not be harmless to the host. If it is, it may not stay that way forever. The issue of harm to the host will arise when efficient spread requires destruction of cells crucial to host well-being and/or when it requires a virus load too high to be handled by host immunity. When we see these viruses harm Asian monkeys, we assume they once harmed their natural African hosts.

Several passages of SIV can increase virulence so that it infects more readily and kills faster. It may assume that continued passage would increase virulence to a point, then reverse the development, resulting eventually in an attenuated virus. This cannot be proved. Whatever their virulence in the past, viruses like SRV and SIV can thrive generation after generation without doing harm to their accustomed host.

When SRV and SIV are faced with insufficient numbers of this host and simultaneously meet an abundant new host. they jump, spread, and cause the eventual death of individuals in the new host population. The fact that SIV or SRV in macaques can serve as a model for AIDS gives us some evidence that SRV or SIV cannot easily spread among Asian monkeys without harming them. But there are SIV strains that cause no harm to macaques whatsoever. We do not knowIt is not known whether their proportion in relation to harmful strains or how either kind would affect macaques in nature because neither would ever encounter macaques in nature. Looking from monkeys to humans, while HIV tends to kill us, HIV-1 has no detrimental effect on about one percent of infected individuals. And HIV-2 has no detrimental effect on about 90 percent of the people it infects. In contrast, HIV-1 spreads strongly in humans compared with the chimpanzee SIV.

Though harmful to humans, it is harmless in chimpanzees in the wild. So far we have no evidence from historical accounts that HIV-2 has ever been more harmful to humans—certainly never as harmful as HIV-1 is today. This suggests that from the virus point of view, the current level of HIV-2 spread is optimally adapted to the local West African environment. This is not to say that under different environmental conditions, such as HIV-2 now meets in India, the virus will not behave differently. Since HIV-2 seems happy with circulation that is not widespread, we must rethink "widespread" from a virus point of view. To us, it has a global connotation, but to a virus, a small area may be wide enough.

Currently, HIV-2 can sustain itself by infecting about one percent of West African humans, especially since SIV provides backup, continually crossing over from West African monkeys to start new strains of HIV-2. This SIV needs little help from its human variant to sustain the family. Monkeys are its main reservoir, and what little is contributed by HIV-2 is incidental to family survival. In contrast, humans are the main reservoir of HIV-1. Though the virus may have come to us from chimpanzees, it appears to be rare in those animals today.

No other host for HIV-1 is known among primates or any other animals. The virus seems to rely for its survival completely on human dissemination, and humans have spread it beyond its original boundaries. Normally it would have remained limited to its original homeland in the western equatorial rain forest, but humans increasingly travel the world. They now carry HIV (and all human pathogens) far and wide. The chances are close to zero that a human virus infection will remain confined to its natural ecological niche, as do the infections of most animals (unless those animals are transported by humans). So HIV-1 might have been happy with circulation in a very local human population, but we ourselves have carried it far beyond its natural evolutionary pathway. Another way to contrast HIV-1 and HIV-2 is to look at their genetic closeness to related viruses.

The SIV of sooty mangabeys is so closely related to HIV-2 that some monkey strains are hard to tell apart from human strains. This means that SIV can shift to a human host as HIV-2 with very limited adaptation, perhaps none at all. The virus can just do its usual thing: when it finds itself in a human, it can replicate without much problem. It reproduces a little less than in a sooty, perhaps, but can comfortably sustain itself. One may say that this SIV is optimally adapted not merely to one species of monkey or primate but to a whole community of human and nonhuman primates. It is adapted to the shared habitat of humans and monkeys in West Africa. Multiple adaptations lead to virus flexibility in terms of hosts, which leads to virus survival at low cost to the population at hand.

The spread of SIV/HIV-2 as well as BaEV argues for this line of reasoning, though SRV offers an exception. SRV is apparently quite comfortable infecting only talapoins, even though humans are handy. It has been noted that the virus load in SIV-infected but healthy sooty mangabeys is as high as the load of HIV-1 and HIV-2 in individuals who are developing AIDS (but much higher than in individuals not developing AIDS). Although this point is still debated in the scientific community, it appears to suggest that the level of circulating virus is indeed related to effective spread, but varies in its effect on the host species. Clearly, the sooty mangabey can remain healthy with an amount of virus in its body that makes humans very sick.

Progression to disease after HIV-1 or HIV-2 infection depends more on our genetic makeup (as a species and as individuals) than the makeup of the virus. Obviously, we would greatly benefit if HIV-2 could outcompete HIV-1 in the human population, but this seems unlikely. Studies conducted in Dakar, Senegal, by the Harvard group headed by Phyllis Kanki and Max Essex show that, under similar conditions, heterosexual spread of HIV-2 is much slower than HIV-1. There data suggest that HIV-2 is less infectious and therefore less capable of maintaining itself than HIV-1 in a human population.

Sexual transmission of HIV-2 is rare, and its perinatal transmission is even more rare compared with that of HIV-1. Since sexual and perinatal transmission are the most common routes in Africa, HIV-2 will lag far behind HIV- 1 in a shared environment on that continent. Not only is HIV-2 slower to infect than HIV-1, but it is much slower to cause disease. In short, in a competitive situation, HIV-1 spreads well and usually makes the host sick. HIV-2 hardly spreads at all and causes disease, if ever, only several decades after infection. An individual is undeniably better off with an HIV-2 infection than with an HIV- 1 infection.

In fact, in places like West Africa, where both viruses circulate, HIV-2 offers some protection against HIV-1. The Kanki and Essex group have shown that individuals infected with HIV-2 are less likely to be infected with HIV-1 than those who are not infected with HIV-2. They found that only after HIV-2 infection has caused a decline in CD_4^+ cells can HIV-1 infection get a foothold. However, this means that HIV-2 protection is only temporary and, once dual infection occurs, disease progression is faster than with either infection alone.

We must remember that HIV-2 is an AIDS virus: it will ultimately cause AIDS and death when it manages to cause infection and disease. Its temporary protection against HIV-1 is nevertheless a good sign. It suggests that a weak AIDS virus has the potential to protect against a much stronger one, even when the two are as distantly related as HIV-2 and HIV-1. Limited evidence pointing in the same direction comes from the rare individuals infected with HIV-1 who are long-term nonprogressors. These are individuals who escape impairment of the immune system for more than ten to fifteen years.

Most of them can thank their own unusually good immune response and/or HIV target cells that are unusually poor at propagating the virus. But a tiny fraction of them (less than half a percent of all individuals infected with HIV-1) must thank their luck in catching an attenuated HIV-1 strain. The big problem is that although attenuated HIVs may protect individuals, such strains are not likely to end the AIDS epidemic by outcompeting the more dangerous HIVs in the general population.

This at least is true of the naturally attenuated strains we have seen so far. Whether HIV-1 or HIV-2, naturally attenuated strains simply do not spread efficiently. To do so, they would have to increase their production. This would probably make them more virulent, putting us back where we started. Is there any way that a retrovirus can spread well while doing its host no damage? We all know the answer by now. It can, but only in the right host. African green monkeys and sootys, as well as talapoins, can cope with high levels of circulating virus without experiencing the slightest sign of harm from their SIV or SRV strains. It seems likely, but cannot be proved, that when these populations were first exposed, most infected monkeys died. If so, a few males and females must have been able to survive infection. They produced offspring also able to survive infection, and eventually the monkey population—the ecological niche—was dominated by hosts that could coexist peacefully with the virus. Another kind of coexistence has been seen among certain mice. The story starts early in this century when researchers developed AKR mice, a strain that is extraordinarily likely to get cancer of the thymus. In the end, this cancer causes the death of virtually all affected mice about a year after birth.

Though discovered in laboratory mice, this intricate phenomenon also occurs in a certain type of feral mouse. In this wild population it is offset by another phenomenon: an intriguing case of retroviral protection against retroviral disease. It was detected in studies by Murray Gardner, Christine Kozak, and Stephen O'Brien of the University of California at Davis and the National Institutes of Health at Bethesda and Frederick, Maryland. In the late 1960s, Gardner captured many types of wild mice in southern California. Testing them for infection with cancer-causing retroviruses, he found most types free of them, but one population was not. Gardner had captured this population on a farm near Lake Casitas. Now called Lake Casitas mice, they were found to be infected with murine leukemia virus (MuLV). Over a period of observation, almost one-third of the animals developed disease: 18 percent had lymphoma and 12 percent had paralysis of the hind limbs. Later two strains of MuLV were identified, one causing the cancer and the other, paralysis. Since the infection rate was so high and about a third of the infections were lethal, long-term survival of the Lake Casitas mouse population was surprising.

Even though MuLV-induced disease occurs only after sexual maturity, the infection and its detrimental effects would be expected to decimate these mice and eventually to wipe them out. This was especially true since MuLV is primarily transmitted by milk ingestion. A substantial proportion of Lake Casitas mice never became infected with MuLV despite its endemicity. This proportion was resistant even to direct injection of purified virus, whereas the rest of the mice were vulnerable.

A virus-host balance had somehow been established in which the virus survived in the vulnerable population (which eventually got sick and sometimes died), while the host population survived in its resistant members. If all Lake Casitas mice were vulnerable, they would eventually die out, taking the virus with them, but virus and host had reached a kind of detente. During more than twenty years of observation, the Lake Casitas mouse population was seen to remain MuLV-infected at a stable level of just over 50 percent. MuLV-induced disease remained the main cause of death among these mice, but the virus did not overwhelm the population. Nor did the number of MuLV-resistant mice grow to threaten virus survival. This story shows that a retrovirus can sustain itself very effectively in a population that is partly susceptible to infection and partly resistant. The virus could sustain itself because it was passaged to the next mouse generation during feeding of the newborns, before disease debilitated any infected mice.

Gardner wondered exactly how the protective phenomenon worked. He found the answer by breeding AKR females with Lake Casitas males with and without MuLV infection. His question was, did mating with a MuLV-resistant male produce offspring resistant to the blood cancer or leukemia seen in all the AKR mothers? The answer was that when the father was completely resistant, that is, he had two MuLV-resistance genes, one on both chromosomes. However, when the gene was resistant but had only one MuLV-resistance gene, the offspring were split. Half were resistant and half were not. What was this gene that protected some Lake Casitas mice against MuLV infection? As we know, a retrovirus enters a susceptible cell because the proteins on the viral envelope can attach to a receptor molecule on the cell surface. The moment cells are infected by a retrovirus, they become resistant to infection by retroviruses that use the same receptor. They are shielded by viral interference since their receptor molecules are saturated with bound envelope molecules.

In the MuLV-resistant Lake Casitas mice, the receptor molecules were found to be saturated. However, no sign of prior infection was seen. The mice were postulated to have an endogenous and crippled version of MuLV that expressed an MuLV envelope on the surface of susceptible cells. And indeed it was finally shown, by Hidetoshi Ikeda and Haruhiko Sugimura of the University of Tokyo as well as by the American group of Christine Kozak, that MuLV-resistant mice carry a truncated and noninfectious fragment of MuLV in all their cells. The bottom line is that, at this point, all Lake Casitas mice are infected with MuLV. About half have the exogenous virus that makes them sick; the others have the endogenous virus that keeps them well.

Apparently, this situation benefits not only the mice but the virus; at least it does not threaten the virus. It shows that optimal host-virus interaction need not lead to the complete harmlessness of the virus in a given host population. It seems to suggest a strategy against AIDS: the genetic engineering of humans to give them endogenous HIV that would express an envelope protein to fool exogenous HIV. Unfortunately, there are major problems with this model. First of all, HIV never infects the human embryo, so it could never become endogenous to humans. Even if it could, the treatment is too laborious (and AIDS already too widespread) to render all humans in the world resistant. If somehow this could be accomplished, we would not be resistant to all possible HIV strains but only to the most typical strains.

Natural selection would then favour a typical strains that could threaten us in new ways. Needless to say, we cannot copy the Lake Casitas model by making only half the world resistant. HIV-1 is in a class by itself. The most dangerous of all AIDS viruses, it was pressured to jump from chimpanzees or colobus monkeys to humans. Its arduous route has involved splitting into subtypes, adapting, and spreading according to whatever conditions it met. By now, some subtypes appear optimally adapted to anal transmission, others to vaginal transmission. Either way, all HIV-1 subtypes eventually cause AIDS, and they do so more rapidly than HIV-2.

HIV-1 appears to have no other major reservoir than humans, and, so far, its optimal spread could be achieved only with virus variants that are ultimately fatal. No rapidly spreading and replicating HIV-1 strains have been identified that do not cause disease.

This indicates that HIV-1 will not become harmless to its human host simply through natural selection for the best-spreading variant.

On the other hand, HIV-1 continues to search for more efficient viral dissemination. It spawns more and more recombinants, particularly in Africa but also in Asia. HIV-1 subtype E, the virus that spreads most efficiently in Asia, is a stable envelope recombinant: a subtype A virus with a new coat. Subtype A appears to mate frequently with subtype C, another variant rapidly spreading in Asia. The virus seems to keep looking for the best configuration of its genes for optimal spread in the human population at hand, by the transmission route at hand. Its search may represent an opportunity for human survival.

Perhaps one of its many recombination events will fortuitously yield a rapidly spreading HIV- 1 that is harmless to us. Unfortunately, no evidence suggests that this lucky event is imminent, or even very likely. Somehow we must push HIV-1 evolution in the right direction. Our best long-term strategy against AIDS is to develop a live vaccine. It must be an HIV-1 strain that is harmless (or relatively so) but spreads well enough in the human population to assure strain survival. It must also outcompete more harmful strains. It must be a strain that can take over and drive HIV-1 into oblivion, as HIV-1 now threatens to do with HIV-2 in West Africa. Such a strain is not likely to occur naturally. We have seen that naturally attenuated HIV strains do not spread well enough to outcompete dangerous strains. We must develop conventional vaccines that consist of HIV proteins, or antigens, that spark our immune system to defend us better. Science will continue to seek treatments that lower the level of virus. Ideally they will not only limit disease in the treated individual but limit viral potential to infect new hosts.

However, we cannot be over-optimistic. Such therapies are on the horizon but will most likely involve drugs that will be far too difficult and costly to provide to the whole world, particularly to the people at highest risk: those living in poor areas without education or health services. Right now, brief treatment of pregnant women can often reduce perinatal HIV infection of newborns. It is not only costly but must be delivered just at the end of pregnancy. A constantly shifting combination of drugs is needed to keep up with shifts in HIV resistance. Even with the best combination, infections will keep spreading, and HIV may well develop multidrug resistance, making treatment harder and harder.

Already drug-resistant mutants have begun to circulate that hamper the two-part goal of reducing disease and reducing infection of new hosts. The conventional type that elicits immunity may never completely prevent HIV infection. However, once infection occurs, such a vaccine could lower the circulating virus load, preventing spread of infection and progression to AIDS. This idea is feasible but, so far, no vaccines consisting of individually produced viral proteins have been tested in humans. Their development has been severely delayed by the lack of an HIV-1 animal model, a living humanlike system in which to observe vaccine effects. Such an animal is still lacking, but we now have the next best thing. Classically, immunity to the all-important virus envelope leads to prevention of infection, or at least disease. Based on this concept, a virus was recently constructed, in the laboratories of Bill Narayan in Kansas City and Joe Sodroski with Norm Letvin in Boston, that wraps the genetic material of SIV in an HIV-1 envelope. Known as SHIV, it is SIV disguised as HIV-1. Passages in monkeys have shown these hybrid viruses to be able to replicate and cause disease. Produced by in vitro fertilization, they are man-made recombinants never found in nature. They have opened the way to test quickly all kinds of viral envelope vaccines for their efficacy in protecting against infection and disease development.

The HIV-1 envelope of these hybrids will be recognized by T cells and antibodies that attach to its distinctive proteins. If a preparation of HIV-1 envelope proteins protects rhesus macaques against infection or disease caused by SHIV, the same preparation most likely will also protect humans against infection and disease caused by HIV-1. We now have the means to find a safe and effective vaccine. We have the methods to monitor the shifting movements of HIV-1 strains. We know which viruses to watch and fear the most: HIV- 1C and E in Asia and HIV 1A and C in Africa. But having a vaccine and knowing where to use it do not automatically get it to the people who need it the most.

Distribution remains a frustrating problem. Regardless of where the AIDS epidemic started, the people now at highest risk are the most deprived in the world. A futuristic solution is to introduce HIV proteins in the food chain. The idea of edible vaccines was pioneered by Charles Arntzen of Cornell University in Ithaca, New York. Such vaccines would be simple and non-threatening. Compliance would be assured since food is familiar, generally welcome, and often crucial for survival. The vaccines would be self-administered by those in need, not administered by outsiders often regarded with fear and suspicion. In collaboration with Arntzen, we have succeeded in producing potatoes that contain HIV proteins.

In fact, their genetic material has been augmented with genes that express HIV proteins. But this is only a start. Such proteins must be expressed at a higher level, and, instead of potatoes, they must be expressed in something like a banana: a food with broad climatic range that is natural to Africa, Asia, and South America; a food that can be eaten without cooking. Then, once the reengineered banana is eaten, the trick is to elicit immune response to the HIV proteins it smuggles into our system. Normally, foreign proteins are tolerated by the digestive tract so we can ingest and absorb nutrients. We would never survive if our immune system saw food as non-self and attacked everything we eat. So how can we get antibodies to attack the HIV proteins in bananas and not bananas as a whole or food in general?

One strategy involves the genetic reengineering of the entire banana plant so that HIV proteins are not only expressed but encased in some kind of toxin. When the fruit is eaten, the digestive system will react to the toxin and trigger an immune response. The rest of the banana will be accepted as usual. But if everything fails, we may still need a living vaccine, an HIV strain that will work for us. This evolutionary path might be our best long-term answer to AIDS. Such a strain, if introduced into a population at risk for HIV-1 infection, might offer individuals protection against HIV-1 and, ideally, would outcompete HIV-1 in the population. But this kind of evolutionary project demands answers to many big questions. First of all, it is not yet certain that the disease-causing effect of HIV-2 can be separated from its efficient spread and replicative capacity. The same is true for HIV-1 strains: all subtypes that spread efficiently appear also to cause disease. Second, though we have SHIV, we still lack an animal model for HIV-1 or HIV-2 as they appear in nature; this is because in nature no other primate or animal of any kind gets sick from HIV infection. Third and most frightening, only vigorous and well-replicating new HIV strains will protect against today's aggressive HIVs—but what if these new strains get out of hand? Can a vigorous and harmless virus be constructed without even the slightest chance of back mutation into a harmful virus?

This living vaccine must also spread from one host to another by sex or some other natural route. If a live, attenuated vaccine strain cannot spread naturally in the global community but can only replicate after injection in the body of a single host, its chances look poor from an evolutionary point of view. It probably cannot outcompete its naturally spreading and aggressive counterparts.

For every man, woman, or child injected with the harmless strain, many more individuals would be infected with the harmful strains. A concerted worldwide effort would be required to vaccinate every single person at risk for AIDS at such speed that the wildtype HIV-1 strains would suddenly find no unprotected humans to infect. The virus must be locked out so abruptly and securely that it has no time or place to adapt for survival.

We must know the AIDS virus very well to tame it, and already our knowledge gives us promising options. But we must recognize that science will find no quick or final solution to HIV or AIDS. Science alone cannot control this virus. Now that the HIV family has found the human family, it will always be with us in some form. All people must know HIV and work to control it. The buying and selling of blood is a highly developed industry in India. Private pathology laboratories collect and pay for blood from individual donors and sell this to hospitals and clinics.

Despite the risks involved in the commercial blood collection system. India cannot afford to stop this practice because about half the blood used in large urban hospitals is obtained in this way. Commercial blood donors are a group particularly at risk of being infected with HIV. The virus can be transmitted through the use of unsterilized equipment in blood collection centres, and also by behaviours such as unprotected sex (both anal and vaginal) with multiple partners.

Contaminated blood can then quickly spread the virus to blood recipients, to the sex partners of the infected person, to other donors (through the use of unsterilized needles), to blood products, and to the foetuses of pregnant women who receive transfusions.

Unsafe sex: some case studies

1.sexual negotiation

The key focus of this study was on how the process of sexual negotiation is carried out at places where men have sex with men and on how men make sense of the sexual encounters they have in such places. As a setting for our study we chose the erotic oases in present day Swedish gay culture; in this case, three video clubs. Other erotic oases are public toilets, parks, nude beaches, sauna clubs, bar back rooms, etc. places that are part of the gay and bisexual subculture found all over the Western world. Our main research method was participant observation. Five male observers with different social and educational backgrounds were trained to make observations and collect field notes in the video clubs investigated. Each observer made approximately 20 visits to the clubs, each visit lasting four to five hours. The observers were recruited from the gay community and were all regular and experienced visitors to different gay subcultural scenes. Since it was considered extremely valuable to obtain as much detailed information as possible concerning all types of sexual negotiations taking place in the milieu, our observers were instructed to act just as they normally did when they visited these places.

As regular visitors, they easily passed as members and they did not have to 'become the phenomenon.' Since they usually did participate in sexual encounters, and since the context in which these took place was what we were most interested in, we did not apply any restrictions on their participation. The only restriction the observers them selves agreed upon beforehand was to accept and engage only in safer sex practices if they were involved in sexual encounters.

Undoubtedly some of the most valuable field notes are derived from those occasions where the observers themselves engaged in sexual negotiations and sexual practices. The notes from these episodes display, in great detail, each step of the negotiation procedure.

Especially valuable here are the observers' own narrative reflections about what they were experiencing in different situations. Within the team, there has been continued scientific debate about what degree of participation in the life and activities to be studied was most adequate. The only thing we can say for certain is that total and total passivity both have their advantages, and participation and total passivity both have their advantages and disadvantages.

Anyone who believes that sex at public toilets is a new invention should listen to the stories hat some of our about the 'glory holes' at some of the city's out houses in the 1940s.

The ideal type of homosexual man who entered the scene in those days was rather effeminate. The gay clubs were members-only clubs, carefully hidden behind locked doors and curtained windows. There was a considerable amount of male prostitution, especially during the Second World War.

With the coming of the end of the 1960s and during the 1970s a different scene took over. Venues such as discos, bars, etc., came into existence which, while still under-ground, but more easy to find, were either openly gay or more or less exclusively visited by gay men and lesbians.

During the 1970s at least 20 gay clubs and bars existed in Stockholm, among them three gay saunas. The image of Swedish Erotica was known all over the world, although most of this pornography was actually produced in the US. The ideal type of gay male in Stockholm in the 1970s was a mixture of queen, the androgynous type of the then dominant youth culture, and the emerging San Francisco 'wannabee butch man.

In Sweden, like elsewhere, the coming of the 1980s meant a drastic change to the more hedonistic gay life-style of the 1970s. Approximately 50 per cent of those who tested HIV positive appeared to be gay or bisexual men.

During the 1980s two major discourses of HIV prevention developed, the safer sex strategy of the gay community, and the more social control-oriented strategy of the responsible authorities. These two discourses have not always found agreement on the right way to handle the HIV problem.

In 1985 the government introduced a new law on infectious diseases which actually allowed the authorities to isolate HIV-positive persons who did not behave.

In 1987, the government introduced a special law forbidding gay saunas. The law was criticized mainly for being a shot in the dark, since men continued to have sex at other erotic oases. It was also criticized for being counterproductive, since it hindered gay organizations in their attempts to implement counselling or HIV prevention at places that could be defined as 'allowing sex on its premises' The law was more a symbolic act of the government than a contribution to real prevention. At the same time the government gave financial support to the Swedish Federation for Gay and Lesbian Rights' (RFSL) new house in the centre of Stockholm. When this—Europe's Largest Gay House' was—opened in 1988, it symbolized the shift from the earlier 'closeted' gay scene to a more open and proud one.

The house has no curtains in its windows. It even advertises itself with neon signs and a bookshop. At the opening ceremony the appearance of prominent cultural and political showed this part of the gay culture had become widely accepted. Furthermore, a parliamentary committee was instructed to investigate the possibility of introducing a law on registered partnership for gay and lesbian couples. The rationale behind this well-intended but contradictory policy of both support and prohibition probably in an attempt by the government to encourage stable relationships among gay men through the establishment of meeting places far away from erotic oases, which were considered to be foci of infection.

In this way public concern was very much directed towards supporting and accepting the 'well behaved' gay men and lesbians while educating the 'badly behaved.' This attitude is very much in line with the old tradition of the Welfare State as a Good Father, who sets life in order for his children. This Father was surprised that some of his children wanted to solve their problems in their own way.

The Father wanted to change the HIV prevention strategy of the gay organizations into a strategy that emphasized testing and contact tracing, and through a large media campaign he at tempted to raise, the awareness of the general population. HIV had to be 'dehomosexualized' in order to fit into the public discourse. Many gay and bisexual men indeed left the scene because of AIDS.

Others visited the oases less frequently; but for quite a few, both younger and older men, occasional sexual encounters still play an important role. Nowadays, however, a drastic change has taken place. Gay and bisexual men generally practise safer sex techniques but obviously not all of them, and not all of the time.

In its role as an erotic oasis the gay sauna has been replaced by, among other places, the video club. It is this scene that we will examine more closely in this chapter. In what follows we will present a description of the cruising patterns at some of these video clubs. Here Erving Goffman's metaphors for social interaction are particularly relevant. There is a striking the social interaction that takes place here and as in a theatre. We perceive actors and an audience, backstage and on-stage and prompters, stage directions and stagehands. The observations for this study were conducted in a number of these clubs, each with its own distinctly different characteristics. One of the clubs describes itself as Europe's largest porno house. It is run by a large porno and sex club company that normally addresses a heterosexual audience.

In this video club you can either watch a movie on three big screens upstairs or you can go downstairs to watch any of the over 60 different pornographic videos that are shown simultaneously in small cabins. The films attract people with diverse sexual tastes; heterosexual, gay, lesbian, bisexual, animal, sadomasochistic, etc. There are about 30 small cabins in the hall and in all of them you can zap between the 60 video channels. The sound, coming simultaneously from all the cabins, is sometimes a total cacophony. Another club has been rebuilt since the law on sauna clubs was introduced in 1987.

In the first room the visitor can watch heterosexual films, in the one farther down bisexual films, and gay films are shown nearest the rear of the premises. This organization of the movies is important. At this video club a more insecure man can start by watching heterosexual films just inside the entrance, then advance to the next room, where he can watch bisexual films, and eventually graduate to watching gay films in the rooms farther down. The visitors to the video clubs have to learn how to use the premises. They have to know whether or not the staff are 'friendly and well disposed.' They have to learn how to find their way once inside the premises. They have to discover what is allowed and what is a 'no, no!' It takes a while for a novice to comprehend all these things. One important part of this game is to be able to distinguish between the hot and the protected areas.

Some parts of the premises are especially hot. Here you are expected and allowed to approach someone sexually. To be present in a certain area of the premises announces one's sexual availability. There are many strategies for responding to different approaches from other actors. And, to make matters more complicated, some of the performances taking place in these hot places are either 'open' to the audience or 'closed.' One of the video clubs is divided into smaller salons where different types of movies are shown. This means that there are some dark corridors or passages between the salons. Certain passages here are very hot. To lean against the wall in one of these passages signals that you are open for suggestions.

Several video clubs have small clubs for- private viewing. These, of course, are also perfect for sexual encounters. If you sit in one of the small cabins with the door slightly open, you are probably putting out a sexual invitation. Some of the video clubs are furnished with two-seater sofas, rather than the normal circles of movie seats. A considerable degree of cultural competence is required to how to sit on these sofas in order to show either or of interest. To sit on one of the two seats with the legs slightly spread is often a sign of availability. To sit in the middle of the sofa 'occupying' both seats is, of course, a sign of inaccessibility. In some video clubs backrooms have developed behind suitably hung curtains in front of emergency exits or some other corners of the premises. These corners may be very hot.

At yet another video club the foyer between the movie rooms and the toilets is regarded as a suitable place for 'asking for a dance,' with a long row of men walking to and from the toilets while eyeing the 'wallflowers' on the sofa. Now and then the men's eyes meet and the man sitting on the sofa strolls after the first man into the toilet. The toilets are hot places. One of the toilets has two rooms and the inner room has a 'glory hole' in the door, probably constructed by a visitor. This place is very popular. Some men hold court there for hours. This is predominantly a place for oral sex. In other places the owners themselves have deliberately built in such services.

Other areas are protected contacts are not expected there, and not allowed. Protected areas function as a refuge for straight men or simply want to take a rest. Others use protected areas more artfully. Sometimes they are occupied by men who seem to be 'straight' but who, with this 'disguise' may actually intend to make themselves even more attractive. After a while a person may move over to the hot places, where he gets some extra attention. Straight men are often highly valued. Persons who close the cabin door at video clubs if there are cabins, of course want to be left free of attention, at least for the time being.

Men who place themselves in one of the rows closest to the screen in the heterosexual salon will probably also be left alone, but may, in exceptional circumstances, be approached by some of the more tenacious hunters. The back rows closest to the aisle are not protected at all against advances from men who are standing behind them trying to catch other men's attention. A certain armchair in the gay film room in one of the video clubs is protected, while a similar armchair farther back closer to the entrance is fairly hot.

Men of all ages, from 17 to 90, are visitors to the clubs. It is somewhat surprising that so many young men find them attractive. Some clubs are obvious 'after hours' places, where you can go after the gay discos have closed. A couple are actually open 24 hours a day. The clubs seem to fulfil a need for initiation —or *rites-de-passage* into gay sexuality for some young men. The gay discos, the organizational gatherings, the bars, are all important places for social activities, and maybe even for searching for Mr. Right. However, some young men seek more uncomplicated ways of having sex in order to get it over with. Most of the visitors to the gay video clubs identify themselves as gay men, but some have told us that they consider themselves to be straight or bisexual; some are married.

The video clubs are first and foremost homo-social milieus. At times some of these men, maybe on their way home after work, or at lunch, cross the border of their sexual identity and engage in an anonymous sexual encounter with another man. This in fact bears many resemblances to male sexual patterns that we can wit ness in many other cultures. Some of the clubs are more gay than others. In some video clubs it is assumed that you are interested in having sex with other men until you have demonstrated otherwise. You are expected to be gay or bisexual. In others it is far more hazardous to make this assumption. Outsiders often ask themselves what attracts men from such different backgrounds to hang around for hours at places where pornographic videos are shown.

Pornographic videos, both heterosexual, bisexual, and gay can he rented for approximately the same price as the entrance fee to the video clubs, and you can keep the movies in your home for 24 hours. The films, of course, are one of the attractions, but they seem to play an astonishingly small role. It isn't even necessary to show gay films. Sometimes places that show al most exclusively straight films are just as attractive as those showing predominantly gay or bisexual movies. It is something else that attracts: the opportunities these places, and other erotic oases, provide for homo-social intercourse and sexual encounters between men. Even if by no means all male visitors fulfil their sexual fantasies with other men, the homo-erotic atmosphere seems to be the most important part of the video clubs' inner life. For some men the clubs serve as a safe place for cruising and for others they also offer a reasonably safe place for quick and often anonymous sexual encounters. It is not only the visitors who participate in the performance. Sometimes it is very difficult to know whether the owners are really aware of what's happening on the premises or not. At one level both the owners and the visitors have a mutual interest in disguising the fact that sexual acts are taking place.

But at the same time it is in the interest of the owners to let the visitors know in a circuitous mariner that they are allowed. Due to the law on gay saunas this is a carefully constructed scene, created by the visitors and the owners of the clubs in cooperation. The aim is to provide space on the premises where sexual acts can take place without revealing this to outsiders. A special cruising script, with its own choreography, has emerged at the video clubs. It is important to note that the performances bear a greater resemblance to a pantomime than to a normal play. The main form of communication consists of nonverbal expressions and movements.

If we ignore a few whispers, and some moaning and whimpering, the only sound heard comes from the somewhat exhausting soundtracks of numerous acts of sexual inter course on the screen. Apart from this, the video clubs are a very good example of Delph's silent community. Not many words were either spoken or overheard during several hundred hours of observation. This is quite different from the pattern common at heterosexual cruising places, like singles bars, where the spoken word is a part of both the cruising and the cooling out strategies. The script tells the visitors how to approach each other in a proper way and the appropriate way of showing interest, or lack of it. The visitors must use a special language in order to present themselves to their coactors and perhaps also to an audience.

The pantomimic dance performed at the video clubs involves following the person in whom you are interested all around the locality, until you get him where you want him, i.e., where you can have sex, or at least where you can negotiate the possibilities in more detail. A man sits on one of the sofas. Another man sits down on the sofa, beside the first man. The first man 'asks for a dance' with a glance, followed by a gentle touch of his crotch. If the glance is met, the man rises and starts walking around in the club to other rooms, watching other films. The second man, if he is interested, follows. The second man may be leaning against the wall close to the first one. The first one moves again with the other, clinging to the first man's 'skirt.' Finally they end·up near the toilets or one of them drifts behind the curtain to the back-room, with the other following, When inside, new dance steps follow.

Now the negotiation is more concerned with the way the two will have sex. Standing in one of the corners of the back-room with your back towards the others and glancing through the tiny slot of the curtain most probably signals that you are interested in passive anal sex, while leaning against the wall most probably signals that you like oral sex or active anal sex. A man who squats on his bended knees is ready to give a 'blow job. Another strategy, mostly seen in the corridors of video club two, is to stand so close to another visitor that you actually rub your own body against the other man's body. If the response is positive there are different alternatives for continuation. A walks over to another room to find out if B is interested. If he is, he follows, not immediately but after a minute. This is repeated a couple of times and in a while the two end up at a place where the sexual act can take place.

One man is leaning against the wall in one of the rather narrow pas sages, at least pretending to watch the movie in the room in front of him. Another man approaches, passing the first man a couple of times to see if he gets any eye contact. The man who is standing still answers the glance and maybe reinforces the sign of interest by placing his hand on his crotch. Then, finally, depending on his sexual preferences, the second man places himself behind the first man or in front of him, squeezing either his penis against the other man's burn or vice versa. Sophisticated strategies have also developed to avoid intimate contacts or to 'turn down' or 'cool out' attentive admirers. Sometimes the fact that someone is actually speaking is a clear indication that there is no point in continuing the complimentary call .

To keep close to friend is another strategy used mainly by the younger men visiting the clubs late at night. Their giggling and whispering keeps admirers at a safe distance, The way one sits in the two-seats sofas is a clear A man sitting in the middle of the sofa covering his crotch with his jacket is probably not very open to sexual invitations. On the other hand also be the starting point of something. The best way to find out is to sit down beside him, trying to make eye contact, and to show your own availability. Maybe he is masturbating furtively inside his trousers. So far this looks like a match. He is open to sexual attentions, but maybe not from the person sitting beside him.

One cool out strategy would be to stop masturbating and fold one's arms demonstratively. Some men sit on the sofas showing their 'weapons.' This is often, of course, a clear invitation and also a 'presentation of the self' and one's phallic merits. But it does not necessarily indicate an invitation. The display of an erect penis while sitting 'on post' can also be an avoiding or even aggressive act, a marker of space and territory. The observers many times witnessed a great hesitation among the men to approach someone in this position. In most gay video clubs you do not risk being caught by anyone oil the staff.

At least two of the clubs are run by gay staff and they do not seem to mind what goes on. So why bother about all those advanced pirouettes, like birds in a courtship dance? Maybe the dance is the main attraction. Or maybe the dance is a necessary part in the complicated process of sexual negotiation between people who are, in most cases, total strangers. The worst thing that can happen at places like this is rejection. If you approach each other step by step and very carefully put your offers and demands on the negotiation table, you will discover at an early stage whether the other person (a) is interested, (b) suits you, (c) is interested in what you are interested in, (d) is willing to have sex here, (e) is interested in having sex the way you prefer it, etc. But the dancing is also a reflection of the long history of repression of same sex behaviour which has forced gay and bisexual men to conceal and disguise their sexual acts both from the authorities and from a hostile environment. This has also forced the men to concentrate on sophisticated rituals for negotiating the act, rather than on the rites of attendance. The aim of the performances is in most cases the sexual act, even though we also see quite a number of 'cock teasers"' who obviously enjoy the dance more than the sexual act itself.

Most of the sexual that take the video Clubs involve masturbation and masturbation approximately 60 per cent of all sexual acts. The second most popular way of having sex here is undoubtedly, oral sex. Like masturbation, it can be performed concealed, in the toilet, or more publicly, behind the curtain, ill the aisles, or even in the sofas and seats. We estimate that approximately 35 per cent of all sexual acts in the video club consist of oral sex. In comparison with mutual masturbation and oral sex, anal sex is rarely practised in the video clubs. This makes up only a few per cent of all sexual acts.

There are very practical reasons for not participating in anal sex in these clubs. Furthermore, there are still many taboos surrounding it, even among men who have sex with men. Since unprotected anal intercourse is the most risky sexual technique for transmitting HIV, anal sex may also have come to be considered even more shameful in recent years, at least if done by publicly. For that reason it is most often practised behind closed doors. However, our observers did witness some acts of anal sex in at least one of the video clubs. The observers witnessed a number of oral acts, which may arguably be labelled safer sex.

The most problematic observation, of course, is the amount of unsafe sex that occurs at places like the video clubs, i.e., predominantly unprotected anal sex. The observers witnessed anal sex a condom used in most of the cases. This is considered to be safer sex. But we also observed cases where persons let themselves be anally penetrated without any protection, which of course is unsafe sex.

There are different strategies for the inclusion of communication about safer sex practices in this dance. Some stopped in the middle of an act when their partner tended to go over the limit, for example, trying to penetrate or be penetrated by the other person. Some handed over a condom to the other partner. Others just put a condom on themselves. There is no need for verbal speech in this manner of communicating, but sometimes a few words were over heard. In most of the cases it was the passive partner who introduced a condom into the negotiation procedure around anal sexual encounters. If the passive partner did not put the condom on the negotiation table, the act was usually an unsafe one. If one partner demanded a condom, the other partner, most often accepted this as a fact of life. No one walked away or interrupted an anal sex act if a condom was introduced. But this did occur in oral sex sessions. The passive partner, in particular the one that sucked sometimes avoided this if the partner introduced a condom. There is obviously a common consent about the use of condoms in anal sex, but not in oral sex. We also noted that when a younger and older man were involved in sexual activities, the younger man often relied on the older to direct the negotiations.

We will use two concrete examples of sexual negotiations to illustrate our reasoning. A tall, slim man in his 30s is standing to the right behind the curtain gazing out over the room through the tiny slot between the curtain and the wall. A couple of older men are also loitering behind the curtain. A man enters the back-room and places himself behind the first man. After a while he places his hand on the first man's behind. The first man stands still and pulls out his penis and starts masturbating. The second man works the first man's jogging pants down to his knees and continues with rather advanced finger exercises. The first man is standing still and picks up what later realised was a tube of lubricant, squeezing out some of the contents into his hand out could hear it and rubs his ass with the lubricant. The second man has now pulled out his prick, but instead of tucking the first man he penetrates him with his fingers. After that the younger man takes from his pocket what must have been a bottle of poppers and inhales a couple of times, and finally leans forward, after which the second man him, for a long time. Several people have gathered around the two, since the younger man is having difficulties keeping his mouth shut, and is groaning quite loudly'. Everybody, tries, in one way or the other to take part and masturbate him, suck him, or stick their finger up ass while he is being fucked. There are approximately five or six persons behind the curtain. A very attractive young person, around 18 to 20, is standing there without moving for a long time.

Nobody seems to dare to court him. Fie reminds me of the beautiful princess who never got the prince because no prince believed that he was good-looking enough. He wears worn out jeans and a white tank top. He leans towards the wall, but takes no initiatives of his own. A man in his 40s, with leather jacket, jeans, and leather boots, finally places himself in front of the young man and soon touches his crotch. He meets with no resistance and his hands continue to touch the young man's body, especially his nipples. The older man is very rough and now and then he slaps the younger man's buttocks. The older man pulls out his penis, pressing the younger man onto his knees, after which the younger starts to suck him. After a while the younger man rises again and starts to kiss the older man. The young one unbuttons his jeans and lets them fall to the floor, turns his back to the older man and more or less 'threads on' to him. The older man cannot possibly have had the time to put on a condom.

In any case the young man didn't do anything to assure himself that his partner was wearing a condom.

Most sexual activities occurring at video clubs cannot be labelled 'safer.' In order to be able to understand the obstacles to safer sex we must not fall back on theories that indicate only individual shortcomings; rather, we must deepen our efforts to understand what it is in the social interaction and in the context where this interaction takes place that affects the outcome of the negotiation. The architectonic structure of the premises can support or counter act safer sex negotiations. If erotic oases like the video clubs offered a safe environment that encourages safer sex, by for instance exhibiting eroticised safer sex messages, this would naturally encourage the men to include safer sex techniques in their sexual negotiations. We saw very few signs of such messages during our field work. Another contextual aspect is the extent to which the pornography shown at video clubs exhibits safer or unsafe sexual encounters. We can only speculate on their effect, but we have noted that there were very few safer sex messages in the pornography shown at the clubs investigated.

2. Study of homosexual risk behaviour

This study is an integral part of the work of Project SIGMA (Socio-Sexual Investigations of Gay Men and AIDS), which is a longitudinal study, of the sexual and social lifestyle of gay and bisexual men in England and Wales. The Project has inter viewed over 1000 men, half of whom have been interviewed four times at intervals of 10 months.

The main aims of the study are to describe the sexual behaviour and lifestyles of gay and bisexual men; to monitor changes in sexual behaviour in relation to HIV/AIDS; to examine attitudes to different sexual behaviours and relationships; to investigate reactions to safer sex practices; and to estimate prevalence of HIV and other viral infections in a non-clinic group of gay and bisexual men. Project SIGMA uses several complementary methods of obtaining information, including: the detailed structured interview in which each respondent is asked for detailed information on sexual history and current practices, numbers of sexual partners, health, mid attitudes towards HIV and safer sex; the sexual diaries, a daily record of sexual activity kept by respondents for a month after each interview; blood and/or saliva samples collected at the interview by trained staff and tested for HIV-1 antibodies and other viral markers; and the postal survey of sexual behaviour, a self-completion questionnaire which appears in the gay press periodically. There are various methods for collecting data for analysis of sexual behaviour, and their merits depend on what is needed from the data. Retrospective interviews and questionnaires are useful for obtaining general and 'memorable' aspects of behaviour, but they are not efficient means of obtaining detailed data that can more appropriately be obtained from the method of sexual diaries.

The main reason for this is that accurate retrospective recall of detailed sexual behaviour is rarely reliable or accurate beyond a few days.' On the other hand, selection bias is higher in the use of diaries than in survey techniques, simply because keeping a monthly diary on a daily basis involves a more prolonged commitment and it is unlikely to be undertaken by those with a very inactive sex life, thus biasing estimates upward.

A further possible drawback is that volunteers may record their behaviour in a way which they expect it should be.

On investigation, these drawbacks seem not to appear, and many results agree with one's intuition and with the data obtained by different methods. At each wave of the investigation, the subject produces a diary of the last week's sexual behaviour in the presence of the interviewer in the context of the ordinary interviews.

This ensures that the diarist understands needs to go into the diary, and also provides indirect evidence of the ability to recall detailed information. At the end, he is given a month diary kit and he returns the completed diary after the month diary form is completed each day and explicit instructions are for its completion. When the completed diary is received back, it is encoded according to a scheme described in Coxon *et al.* 1992, summarised, and then entered into a database for subsequent analysis.

The chief methodological advantages of the diary method are its ease and flexibility:

(a) it is naturalistic;

(b) it is easily adapted to record sexual data from those of any sexual orientation;

(c) it can be augmented to obtain other concurrent information; and

(d) it can be expanded to take into account such aspects as coital position.

There are a number of more substantive advantages of the diary method:

(a) it allows the detail of sexual behaviour to be recorded and analysed, and to be encoded intact, since the researcher knows the context of any sexual act location, the actors, the adjuncts to sex, and is able to place their use in the correct context;

(b) uniquely, it permits the analysis not only of individual behaviour but of the 'volume' of behaviour, where the denominator is all the sexual acts involved;

(c) it allows sequences of sexual activity to be analysed. Sometimes this can be crucial, for we need to know whether unsafe behaviour tends to occur at the start, middle, or end of a sexual session, and the meaning of acts such as anal intercourse can be substantially different when it occurs as an end-marker rather than as an incidental activity; and

(d) it allows issues of power or dominance in sexual behaviour to be investigated by systematically encoding the modality of the act and thus allowing gendered distinctions to be made between reciprocated and dominance sessions the former where the other partner tends to do the same thing in return to his partner, the latter where one partner is repeatedly the submissive, the other the dominant partner.

The analysis of two aspects of sexual and especially anal intercourse: the effect of relationship type on sexual behaviour and behavioural progression in a sexual act. Before proceeding further, it is important that the reader understand the basics of the system of encoding the structure of sexual behaviour that we have developed, since the results in the tables make use of it. Essentially, every diary is encoded into a database from which application programs may analyse the results.

The encoding process, simply translates the respondent's description of sexual behaviour into a structured formal language that readily lends itself to computer representation. Every diary pack has a preliminary face-sheet eliciting information on HIV status, relationship type, geographic location, etc., in the form of a few preliminary questions, together with a table for the respondent to list sexual partners who are involved in their sexual transactions.

The characteristics include demographic and descriptive information about each partner,' and the list is built up as the diary progresses. They are instructed to enter the time and date, then to describe in normal language precisely what they did, according to a provided set of criteria .

Each such spatially and time-limited sexual encounter is referred to as a session and may involve one or more persons. Each session forms a separate record in the database. The sexual session is subdivided into sexual acts, each of which is finally described by the behaviour and its modality and by its outcome basically whether and how and where ejaculation occurs.

To aid understanding, take the following simple example of a sexual session:

Session: = {PW AS AF}

This session consists of three acts. The first character of each act is the modality., and any remaining characters are the behaviour. The behaviour describes what is done, and the modality does it, There are five modalities, which define who and to whom the diarist's point of view, Ego's partner is referred to as Alter. A comment is in order about the 'H' modality.

Although Ego is not directly in this modality, what his partner does by himself may have possible consequences for HIV transmission, such as when Alter masturbates himself and ejaculates over Ego. At the simplest level, information can be obtained from respondents' diaries to match commonly used interview-based variables such as information referring to the prevalence and incidence of various sexual activities. In interviews, this is obtained by asking the respondent him/herself to estimate how often a given sexual act has been engaged in during a specified period In the sexual diaries such information is derived post factum by the researcher by counting how often a given activity occurs in the diary script. The first area of interest is to see how figures derived from sexual diaries compare at the aggregate level to interview responses.

The more interesting point concerns active and passive variants of sexual behaviours. In a stable and closed the figures for active, and passive variants of a sexual behaviour should be identical. In fact, the figures are surprisingly close to equality, and there is no tendency for there to be more active diarists than passive diarists, as one might expect."

For sexual diary data the differences are smaller than the data from any other method, indicating their greater validity. How similar are these diary data to aggregated self-report data obtained by the interview method?

At first sight and looking at the actual percentages, they are rather different, with some major discrepancies: the rank-order correlation is modest (p= 0.77). More interestingly, the Pearsonian (linear) correlation is much higher (r 0.95), and the regression equation:

Y (estimated interview percentage) = 15.82 + 0.94X (diary percentage)

reveals that the relationship is close to absolute, but with an constant of about 16. That is, if the diary data are more reliable, then the interview method systematically overestimates the incidence figures but keeps a virtually identical profile. One possibility is that in the interview respondents actually use an interval greater than one month and correctly remember having done X, but have done it in a longer period.

A vast majority of gay men's sexual activity is taken up by the three main behaviours of masturbation, fellatio and anal intercourse. The justification for this statement is clearly seen in diary analysis, where the act can be used as the unit of counting. This is termed 'analysis of volume' in our account and is a mode of analysis only feasible using the diary method. Table 1 ilustrate the proportions which various sexual behaviours occupy. In fact, over

80 per cent of all behaviour in the sample consists of these three main activities: masturbation, fellatio, and anal inter course.

Table 1

Sexual Behaviours as proportion of Total Sexual Acts

Behaviour	Frequency of acts	Percentage of total
Masturbation	20,976	58.3
Fellatio	5,990	16.7
Anal int. (F)	2017	5.6
Frottage	1683	4.4
Deep kissing	1346	3.7
Ano-digital insertion	1057	2.9
Massage	921	2.6
Anilingus	813	2.3
Inter-femoral frottage	460	1.3
Corporal punishment	269	0.8
Nipple Play	148	0.4
Ano-brachial insrtion	133	0.4
Vaginal intercourse	126	0.4
Lindinism	39	0.1
Cunnilingus	7	0.02
Total acts	35, 981	100%

Masturbation is by far the most common activity and accounts for three-fifths of the total outlet, with Solo Masturbation accounting for over one-third of all sexual acts. The low figure for DK (deep kissing) is simply a reflection of the fact that most diarists don't consider it to be a sexual act, and therefore don't record it consistently.

The next 16 per cent of sexual outlet is distributed between BR (frottage), DK (deep kissing), FG (digital-anal insertion), MA (massage) and RI (anilingus). Expressed in terms of the total sexual outlet for the group, heterosexual activity (vaginal intercourse (VF) and cunnilingus (CN)) is indeed. Within the diaries, sexual relationship are, defined, following the SIGMA conventions, as:

(a) one regular partner ('closed');

(b) one or more regular partners and others and

(c) no regular partner.

Each of these relationship types is subdivided into three age ranges. Each cell of the resulting ninefold design is given a label, in the form of a roman numeral, as shown in table 2. Patterns of sexual behaviour can then be studied by looking at how the sexual outlet of each of these nine types differs. This is done by treating that type's total sexual outlet as 100 per cent, and then looking at how it is divided between the three most common sexual behaviours and' their associated in modalities.

Table 2

SIGMA Typology: Relationship by Age Types

Relationship	Age		
	Under21	21 to 39	Above 39
One regular partner	I	II	III
Regular partner and others	IV	V	VI
No regular partner	VII	VIII	IX

The behavioural characteristics for each type are well defined:

— *Masturbation.* Those with no regular partner show a very high incidence of solo-masturbation, whereas those in closed relationships have a very low incidence.

— *Anal intercourse.* Those with no regular partner show the lowest incidence of arty form of anal intercourse, with most of their values being significantly less than the 'average' figure indicated in the ALL column. Those in closed relationships show a consistently higher level of both active and passive anal intercourse. Active anal intercourse.

— *Fellatio.* Fellatio seems to transcend the relationship limits, and does not show any consistent relationship pattern. Types IV, V, and 'VI have the highest figures for fellatio, but we should bear in mind that type, IV is by far the smallest set, and so we cannot treat the result as reliable. No other form of behaviour exhibits a significant relationship type or age dependency.

Anal intercourse is recognized as the form behaviour that is implicated most significantly in the transmission of HIV. From a behavioural point of be interesting to see what types of behaviour are most likely to precede an lead on to anal intercourse of some form. Anal intercourse is most typically the end-marker of session and the sequence in a sexual session may be so constrained that anal intercourse becomes virtually inevitable.

Moreover, different behaviours may precede the active as opposed to the passive variant. In a preliminary analysis of the co-occurrence of sexual acts it was found that the two acts most likely to occur in the same sexual session as anal intercourse are masturbation and fellatio. Starting with this, precedence analysis was then applied to the sessions to see what behaviour is most likely to lead on to anal intercourse. Precedence analysis is essentially a frequency count of how many times a given act precedes another in a sexual session.

The analysis uses a 'sensitivity' parameter called 'width' which defines how many acts are, taken into consideration by the analysis as, preceding the reference act. For example, consider the following session:

Session 1: = {AW PW PF AS}

The AS is ignored in a precedence since the reference. If the width is one, then only PW is counted as the precedent, but if the width is 2, then both PW and AW counted as precedents. Thus the width, value defines how acts are visible to the analysis previous to the reference base. But the same act can occur more than once in a session, and this has to be allowed for. Consider the following example:

Session 2: = { AFI AS PW AS AF}

If AF is the reference base, then the three (distinct) precedent are, AFI, AS, and PW. But AS occurs twice, and is therefore given a higher precedence value. In the above example, the precedence value of AS has a value of 2 if the width is 3, but a value of 1 if the width is 2, the reason being that the second AS is out of the range of width visibility when the width is 2. Let us turn now to the diary data. Looking at both the Active and Passive tables, the rank order of likely precedence is the same, independent of the width of the precedence. Active/ insertive anal intercourse is most likely to be preceded (in order) by:

(Passive Sucking/Receptive Fellatio)

(Active Sucking/ Insertive Fellatio)

(Active Wanking/Masturbation), and

(Passive Wanking/Masturbation)

This can be expressed as a rule: 'If fuck a guy, sticking is most likely to precede it. Passive/ receptive anal intercourse, by contrast, is most likely to be preceded by:

(Active Sucking/ Insertive Fellatio)

(Passive Sucking/ Receptive Fellatio)

(Passive Wanking/ Masturbation), and

(Active Wanking/ Masturbation)

A 'successor analysis' of active and passive fellatio would reveal the similar point: 'If you suck your partner, you're likely to go on to be fucked by him,' and 'If you are sucked by your partner, you are likely to be expected to go on to .fuck him. If anal intercourse occurs in a sexual session, then it is most commonly the end marker, and is very likely indeed to result in ejaculation, so this is where attention needs to be focused for a more accurate knowledge of how risk occurs. But this is another story. The results given by the diary analysis are very reliable and conclusive when studying the behaviour of individuals at the session level.

Because of the short of the diaries, it is not so effective for time-generalized analysis, It does, however., give a good idea of relative proportions of outlet sets may be analysed by various independent. The greatest strengths of diary analysis, and areas in which it is particular further study, are, in the analysis of the volume of sexual behaviour of sexual, role segregation, and co-occurrence, precedence, and successor are all methods used to study behaviour at the session or level.

The use of condoms during sessions is also all important part of the study, and one area in which diary analysis can, in principle, perform well. Perhaps the most striking difference is that data are derived in the case of diaries, whereas data represent subjects' accounts in the case of interviews. There is no warrant for believing that the two will necessarily give rise to the same conclusions.

But it is clearly seen front this analysis that sexual diaries are capable of providing unique data which is also uniquely adapted to answering problems of considerable epidemiological and policy relevance. In the research reported here, sexual diaries have been used as an auxiliary method of data collection and validation within a Western European context. The reliability and utility of diaries in other con texts depends on a number of factors: Whether diary-keeping is an accepted procedure in the culture. For gay men, and for sexual and romantic activity in general, diary-keeping is a popular, though often a private, pastime, and is often written in code to ensure confidentiality . The social science use consists primarily in persuading respondents to do so for scientific purposes.

Anonymity must be guaranteeable. Whilst some diarists care not who knows their secrets, for others the diary records what no one else knows, and somehow the social scientist has to safeguard this secrecy, especially if the matters being recorded are illegal, deviant, or even simply private. At least one SIGMA diarist was expelled from his lodgings because his landlady 'found' his sexual diary. The diary does not depend on a written format. Although diaries are most conveniently kept in writing in literate cultures, there is no reason why they must be. We have used both tape recorders and electronic pocket memos to record their diaries. The diary does not depend or a long period. Although we have found that a month is the minimum period for reliable data, some diarists can be persuaded to keep it for much longer.

Card versions of day entries can be devised which allow an encrypted version of events to be sent through the mail on a daily basis, thus avoiding problems of partial completion and loss; it also helps avoid contamination due to recognition of trends by the diarist, if this is felt to be a problem. The diary can be completed at leisure communicating about sexual behaviour is often not feasible or is subject to systematic bias if elicited the presence of others.

Diaries can be completed at any time convenient to the respondent. Diary information can as well be based on observation as on the subjects report. Although, not always the structure of sexual behaviour underlying the diary code makes it possible to use it as a rapid shorthand for situations such is immediate re-interview, and our current studies of competent encoders' encodings of a common video stimulus show that high agreement on 'chunking' and description of sexual activity can be achieved. The sexual diary is a robust, easy-to-use method for collecting re ports on detailed and sequential aspects of sexual behaviour. So long as common meanings are established be fore its use, respondents find them straightforward and even interesting to complete, and the data can be used to answer questions which interviews based on retrospective recall are ill-adapted to answer.

Probably the most telling shortcoming is that volunteer bias is likely to be strong including the earlier point about the difference in diary-keepers. This can be minimized by careful strategies to improve participation. Because of the inherent detail of the diary account, it lends itself to serendipitous discovery and since it provides a general trace of behaviour it can provide well-adapted information if new foci of research become imperative.

3.Study of high risk behaviour

In the beginnings ithe spread of HIV/AIDS was believed to be confined to homosexual men, and indeed was represented as being somehow peculiar to so-called 'gay sex' as if heterosexuals never have more than one sexual partner and never engage in anal intercourse. The early association between the incidence of this disease and certain kinds of sexual behaviour, notably 'deviant' sexual behaviour, resulted in an enormous expansion in the study of sexual behaviour.

A substantial part of virtually every dollar that is spent in AIDS prevention research, even in areas in which drug injection is prevalent, includes an examination of some aspect of sexual behaviour. One would think that nearly ten years later, after the expenditure of tens of millions of dollars, that we would have acquired a clearer under standing of the nature of the sexual behaviours that are associated with the spread of this disease.

Minimally, one would expect that we would at least have a better understanding of what the questions ought to be, and how to best go about trying to resolve them. It is the thesis of this chapter, however, that we are not much closer now to understanding how to foster sexual risk reduction than we were ten years ago.

Indeed, the discussion which follows is aimed at showing how we have been asking the wrong questions about sexual risk behaviour and often, asking them in a manner that is ill-suited to the complex nature of the behaviours themselves. In some sense, the latter methodological problem is antecedent to the former, which might be said to be more fundamentally conceptual in nature, and so that is where the discussion begins. Data bases on high-risk sexual behaviour have been amassed over the last ten years, much of this information remains difficult to interpret, and much of it is of very limited utility in fostering sustained changes in sexual behaviour.

Particularly problematic is the fact that much of this research has employed rather narrow theoretical paradigms in which sexual behaviour is often used as the independent variable. This often ignores any substantial consideration of the broad diversity in gender roles and meanings that exist, or of the way in which both behaviour and meaning are shaped by interacting cultural, social, economic, and political factors. As Carrier and Bolton have pointed out:

> "The usefulness of most AIDS-related studies of human sexual behaviors conducted since the epidemic began is limited because of the narrow range of methods employed to gather data."

This study does not permit an exhaustive treatment of the various kinds of methodological problems that attend contemporary sex research, particularly those which are specific to the study of risk behaviours associated with the transmission of HIV infection.

However to give a couple of from my own ethnographic work, which rate the lack of utility of the kinds of conceptual categories that underpin most survey research on risk behaviour and AIDS, They also highlight the dire result stemming from the use of these categories, for both our understanding of the spread of this disease and to develop appropriate education.

Story of Tina, an Asian-American who is approximately twenty years of age. Born a biological male, at the age of nineteen Tina initiated a process of making herself into a 'female' including breast implants and regular female hormone injection. For several years prior to this, and reportedly since puberty, Tina had dressed as a female and used, what she and others around her commonly identified as 'effeminate,' speech patterns, Indeed, Tina divided her life history into two major parts, her childhood a time that she described as 'before I became a woman' and her early adolescence 'when I knew I wanted a man,' a desire that she identified as consistent with her female gender identity.

Her life story narrative is filled with descriptions of her body, including what she imagines herself to have looked like at various times in her life. Indeed, the way she imagined her body was as if it contained a /woman inside.' It is noteworthy that this also referred to her 'social skin', since she did not identify as homosexual. 'It's not a gay thing,' explained Tina, 'I'm all woman.' This concept of self was consistent with her social behaviour. At the time of her interview in 1989, she was partnered with Roberto, a white, biological male of about the same age. Roberto was, by his own description, a heterosexual male who strenuously denied being involved in any same-sex activity.

Over the course of more than a years' ethnographic observation, including a prolonged period of time of in Tina was away in prison, Roberto was involved in several relationships, all of them biological females. This was so even though, in outward she resembled many of them, 'worked' a similar area in the prostitution stroll on the Lower West Side of Manhattan, was involved in similar sexual behaviours and in fact had many of the same 'johns' as other cross-dressing, trans-gender individuals in this street scene. Finally, and again consistent with her concept of self, it is noteworthy that most of her close social relationships were with heterosexual females. Despite the fact that she openly identified the kind of sex work in which others around her were involved as risky for AIDS, Tina did not believe that she was at risk. She associated risk with 'being gay,' and concluded that since she was not gay, she was not at risk.

The early misre-presentation of AIDS by the medical community as a 'gay disease', and a continuing predilection to employ stigmatizing gender categories that fail to distinguish between issues of sexual identity and issues of sexual behaviour, pro mote such concepts of risk. At the very least, they fail to correct them, often with dire results. About a year later, Tina tested positive for HIV infection.

Another example is the the case of Toni, a Hispanic female, now in her late thirties. Toni came to New York City from Puerto Rico when she was about ten years of age, and lived with an aunt in East Harlem. She found English difficult and had consider able trouble in school. This, coupled with the fact that the household in which she was living could not really support her, eventually led her, around the age of 13, to get involved in street prostitution. She explained that a male friend took her to midtown Manhattan where he hustled, suggesting that Toni, who at the time had very 'boy-like' body features, could probably 'pass.' Recalls Toni, 'He told me, most of them just want blow jobs; it's easy.' Toni was able to pass and, for several years, worked on weekends as a 'male prostitute' in the Times Square area of Manhattan, while continuing in a heterosexual relationship with her boyfriend in Harlem. She was popular on the streets, and in fact was able to don the role of 'chicken' far longer than many of her male counterparts, some of whom she says did not know that she was female and heterosexual. The money she carried made a substantial contribution to her aunt's household.

Like many of her male counterparts oil the streets, Toni was engaged in oral sex and occasionally receptive anal inter course. Nevertheless, she did not see herself as being at: high risk for HIV infection, principally because she regarded herself as female and heterosexual. As Toni became older, however, she found it increasingly difficult to pass as a male. In addition to her high voice and lack of facial hair, she had also 'breasts, Moreover, around this time she became pregnant, y by a boyfriend. After the birth of h er baby, she once again found herself in need of money.

Now several years older, and still without the education and training necessary to obtain a job, she returned to prostitution, this time as a 'woman.' Initially she supplemented her income from Public Assistance by working oil the Lexington Avenue 'stroll'. With strikingly attractive physical features, she was again very popular among the 'johns,' and for a time was able to establish a regular clientele that she 'serviced' on a scheduled basis in her own home. She believed that she was at higher risk for AIDS at this time than in earlier stages in her life. However, her reasons for believing this stemmed largely from the identity of her clients, whom she described as 'junkies,' rather than from a concern about risk from sexual behaviour, per se. Indeed, she told a story about a very well paying customer who was often unable to achieve an erection, a fact that made her wonder if he was 'half gay,' and whether or not he might give her AIDS.

The sexual orientation of the person with whom Toni was engaged in sexual intercourse, either men who have sex with men or men who have sex with women, was irrelevant to her concept of self. As she described it, 'It's just like the guy at the newsstand.... He sells all these male porno magazines.... That doesn't make him gay... It's just business.' Note the difficulty and misconceptions that arise when information about risk behaviour is forged in gender categories that focus attention on is risky, rather than on what is risky. As an adolescent, and in the context of oral sex, Toni that she was safe she because she was not gay.

Later and in the context of high-risk vaginal sex, she acknowledged that she was at greater risk but for the wrong reasons. Her perception of greater risk not from the nature of the specific sexual behaviours involved but rather was a consequence of the social identity of her partners. Indeed, she later described how she was eventually able to move out of street position by setting up a 'private house' out and er pick and by extension, who she had sex with. It is noteworthy that the criteria she described were largely social and economic in character.

Condoms were used only when she thought she was at risk of becoming pregnant, and often not even then 'if the money was right.' Some of the issues and obstacles that the existing approaches to AIDS prevention research are inadequate to address, particularly as they relate to sexual minorities and individuals involved in survival sex. They also demonstrate the way that a failure to distinguish between sex and gender may serve as a substantial barrier to acquiring the kind of understanding of risk behaviour that is critical to the development of effective prevention messages and strategies.

Clearly, if we are to reach sexual minority groups with meaningful and effective HIV/AIDS prevention efforts, we must challenge the use of categories that serve to obfuscate the nature of risk. As Shedlin, Clatts, and Carrier have pointed out in reference to sexual categories in AIDS prevention research: None of the labels provides any real insight or understanding into the complex gender identity issues or range of sexual and drug behaviors which place these individuals and their clients/partners at risk for HIV infection.

In terms of the development of prevention education materials for example, it can be seen that most have little relevance or appropriate advice or backup for biological males who identify as females, and who survive in an environment which seeks unsuccessfully to classify them by a whole range of mutually exclusive labels and terms. These examples also underscore the inadequacy of the rigid and often static clinical and behavioural categories that implicitly super impose some set of biological properties onto sexual behaviour and experience, independent of the processual factors in which these acts occur or the larger sociocultural contexts in and by which they are signified, Rigid categories, such as 'heterosexual,' 'homosexual and even 'bisexual' take sexual activity and sexual identity out of time and place.

The use of these categories makes it impossible to identify and map changes in concepts of self over the course of an individual's life span, or to locate an ever-emergent self within social, cultural, and economic institutions that are themselves dynamic in character. Far from serving to clarify the import of social, economic, and political institutions on risk behaviour, this kind of approach to the study of sexual risk results in the production of enormous bodies of behavioural data, which, because it is devoid of any substantive attention to issues of time and place, is of very limited utility in the development of AIDS prevention strategies.

Of particular concern here are the economic forces that underpin risk behaviour and that may represent acute barriers to risk reduction. Even those studies that acknowledge the systemic economic in equities that persist M these utilize this information for little more than descriptive purposes. Typically these conditions are held as constants, and dubious academic constructions, such as 'self efficacy' and 'locus of control,' are used to explain variance in behaviour. These same dubious entities then become the target for intervention, again with little or no attention to the structural conditions which give rise to perceptions of self, or to those that recreate these systems of power.

Identification of those specific sexual acts that most efficiently facilitate the transmission of HIV was certainly an important break through in the early formulation of AIDS prevention information. The problem in terms of the application of this information is that we have never really got beyond a focus on who puts what part of their anatomy into what part of a partner's anatomy, with or without a condom, and on how many occasions, information that has proven to be largely irrelevant to understanding either the nature of sexual relations or how to foster sexual risk reduction

One of the reasons that rigid sex categories have proven to be so inadequate is that this kind of approach to the study of sexual behaviour has the result of removing behaviour from the socio-cultural institutions in which it is embedded and to which it gives. Take, for the case of Jake, a 23-year-old white male who has been for the past nine years. Born in

Massachusetts, adopted an orphanage at the age, of three, he lived with his adopted and sister in a small town in Maine until he ran away for the very last time at the age of fourteen. He describes his early childhood as one filled with material but plagued with physical and sexual abuse. His father began raping him when he was Only five years old, and his mother, while aware of the situation, did nothing to stop it: 'They didn't know how to treat a child....My father's excuse was that he never had a father to know how to have a kid or be a father.... My mother's was that she wanted to believe that things like that couldn't really happen.' Jake first began running away from home for short periods of time at the age of 10. He used to go over to a friend's house to hide but knowing he couldn't hide forever, he would call up his parents and ask to go home: 'He'd come pick me up, and I'd go back. He'd get me into the bedroom and that's it. Finally, I got sick of him beating me and using me. Jake made his way to Portland, Maine and was forced to fend for himself. He recalls learning quickly that he had something other people wanted, that he was a commodity Since that time he has travelled across the United States, from Maine to California; has been in and out of jail for robbery, possession of drugs, prostitution, breaking and entering, and assault; and has been in and out of hospitals, rehabilitation programmes, and temporary adolescent and adult residences. He takes pride in his ability to survive against the odds but he recalls that 'hustling became serious work' when he became 'a drug addict.'

Says Jake: As an addict, nothing else seemed to matter besides securing the next hit. When you first start, you set your limits. When I wasn't getting high, forty to fifty dollars just to blow me. When I started getting high, twenty bucks to blow me. Then, when I became an addict, my life changed. Five dollars for anything. Anything. Fucking me any thing! You do it just for the next hit. That's when you don't love yourself anymore. Looking back, jake recalled a time in which he thought that hustling was fun, but then it became a job. It's Eke a job. I stand out there from eight at night until four in the morning, selling my ass! That's not fun. It's not fun. It's work!... And the people, they treat you like shit, They don't care about you,. All they care about is getting their nuts off. And sometimes, after they grab you and touch you, they don't want to give you nothing for it. That's not fair, if they touch you they got to, pay for it. It's a job to have. It destroys you. You get old fast. In the last three years he has had many of the opportunistic infections associated with AIDS, and his life is a daily struggle to manage intermittent episodes of diarrhoea, oral upper respiratory ailments, and seizures. His last severe bout of pneumonia cost him a lung and doctors warn him that the next attack might be his very last.

Despite it all, Jake continues to hustle around 'rimes Square and West Village areas of Manhattan. He says that 'business' has been slow lately, and lie attributes this to the fact that he's started to look sick, and word has got out that he has AIDS. Sometimes, he admits, he's able to use this AIDS-thing' to his advantage. Some tricks, upon taking him home and learning from Jake that he has AIDS, give him money just to go away. On most nights of the week, and in all kinds of weather, he can be found on the same corner of a Greenwich Village street, hustling for his next hit. Bitter and withdrawn, he stands on the corner watching the traffic, trying to make eye contact with drivers stopping at the traffic light, eye contact that will signal potential interest. He works all night, earning a few dollars a lime for sex in a doorway' in a parked car, or in the apartment of a mar, whose name he does not know.

By four o'clock in the morning he will have earned enough money to stay high on crack, and even, enough to keep from getting dope-sick the next morning Over and over again, Jake has been told by health care providers that in order to get help 'he to do his share'—a poignant phrase for the kind of supply-side economies that engenders poverty and homelessness. Poignant also for what it says about some of the fundamental assumptions that underpin much of AIDS prevention practice.

The share that Jake is able to do is quite limited. Limited not by his intelligence, his creativity, or his dreams, but rather by his ability, any child's ability, to grow and mature in a world in with his value is subject to the vagaries of the street meat market. As this brief case study reveals, it is of paramount importance that we begin looking more carefully at the way in which high-risk sexual behaviour is embedded in systems of economic exchange, particular of exchange that typify many poor communities in both industrial and nonindustrial world.

For quite apart from the information an individual possesses about risk for HIV transmission, or an individual may perceive as necessary ill order to avoid it or indeed what an might wish to do in order to avoid it a number of complex constraints may serve as overwhelming barriers to an capacity to engage consistent risk reduction. Most of the people in the world ill be at risk for AIDS in the coming decade, are at risk not because of a lack of knowledge, belief, or intention, but rather because of the larger social and economic circumstances that govern their lives. Most will be subject to economic inequalities that have disparities of power and wealth at their core inequalities exacerbated by factors of race, gender, sexual identity.

Hence and this is evident from the study of many other disease outcomes as well economic constraints are a fundamental barrier to arresting the spread of this disease Unfortunately, very little of the current research that is being done' on sexual risk behaviour acknowledges the import of systemic poverty on sexual risk behaviour. Moreover, research paradigms that continue to place a premium on the study of behavioural frequencies and dubious notions of motive are unsuited to the task of identifying ways in which to foster 'actionable' changes in high-risk sexual behaviour. Certainly this fact reflects a failure of political will, but it should also call into question the kinds of priorities that have been established in the AIDS prevention research industry

To continue to pretend that a two hour session with an AIDS educator, for example, can measurably increase 'self-esteem' in a person who has lived an entire lifetime in a context of violence, discri-mination, and abject poverty, or that the problem of 'empowerment 'lies solely in convincing the subject that he or she has power, regardless of whether this is the case, is to completely miss the mark about why people engage in risk behaviour.

At the very least, the assumption that these kinds AIDs is based upon a particular kind of intellectual fiction. Such models hold the conditions in which the subject lives, as well as the factors that have brought him or her to these circumstances, as an analytic 'constant'. It is precisely the force of the social and economic conditions in which an individual lives and works, what Schoepf has referred to as the 'political ecology of disease,' that will in large measure determine why some individuals, rather than others have a substantially greater likelihood of becoming infected.'

Clearly, an individual living in conditions characterized by poor nutrition, inadequate shelter, and ineffectual health care, all of which contribute to poor immune response, will be more vulnerable to developing opportunistic infections than someone who is not confronted by these kinds of circumstances.

Linguistic perspectives of HIV /AIDS

Speakers of English use language in special ways when they talk about the AIDS pandemic and its effects on their lives. They draw on code words and phrases when identifying HIV illnesses, describing symptoms, and assessing treatment strategies. They ad just word order, disguise subject reference, and make other changes in sentence and paragraph form when discussing high-risk behaviour or commenting on the social conditions which encourage risk talking. Sometimes, when AIDS is the topic under discussion, people explore their thoughts and feelings in great verbal detail; other times, they make, their thoughts and feelings known by saying nothing at all.

All discussions of AIDS are rule-governed speech events. What speaker, understand about the pandemic and its effects on their lives helps them choose the features of grammar and discourse which are relevant to, the messages they want to convey in such settings. Frequently, such closely meshed relationships between language and experience create formidable barriers to AIDS education and out reach efforts. As a linguist, my entry point in this research is text-specific instance of conversation, narration, question asking and answering, or other forms of situated discourse. Texts are not arbitrary linguistic phenomena. Text form as well as text content reflect speaker decisions regarding what should be said on the issues being addressed within that speech setting.

In other words, texts can be studied as intentional constructions, and as context-specific products of choice-making. The evidence of intention and choice displayed within each text provides access to the speaker's const-ruction of context-specific messages and to the larger discourse of which those messages are a part.

Frequently, text-centred research confirms claims about AIDS discourse which ethnographers have developed through analysis of other types of social data. And in the process, such research often shows how widely attested features of discourse take on particular significance within the speaker's presentation of message and meaning in specific social domains. In some cases, text-centred research provide a basis for criticizing and working claims about discourse from non-linguistic data sources. During the earliest years of the AIDS pandemic, the biomedical characteristics of what were later to be termed HIV illnesses were puzzling to many people and the social implications of these conditions was the absence of agreement regarding the appropriate name for these phenomena.

In the main, practitioners favoured terms like gay related immune deficiency (GRID), community acquired immune deficiency syndrome (CAIDS), or gay bowel syndrome, labels which 'identified the disease by whom it hit rather than what it did. Acquired immune deficiency syndrome (AIDS) came into use in 1982 and quickly replaced older, more targeted references.

But as, AIDS became an accepted reference for the condition, so did the notion of groups and the identification of forms of behaviour male co-sexual erotics, intravenous drug use) which were most likely to place persons within situation; of risk.

As Clatts and Mutchler have noted, such designations draw explicit connections between AIDS and the 'dangerous and 'other connections which become problematic for AIDS research and education because they 'fix our attention on a relatively small range of possible vectors of this disease... and direct our attention away from other possible factors of (its) aetiology and spread.

These connections between AIDS, danger, antisocial behaviour, and the other have real implications for the grounding of AIDS discourse in context-specific text construction. The terms risk and at-risk are anything but neutral in their suggestion of deliberately unobserved restraint. The term AIDS itself is heavily marked for irregular reference, given the connotation of its headword (syndrome), the ambiguity of its key modifier, and the length or the unabbreviated construction.

The use of the abbreviation intensifies this sense of irregularity by ring the presence of these meanings within sentence structure, Other vocabulary used in AIDS-related text-making Whether they come from the medical discourse on sexually transmitted diseases (STDs) or are derived through analogy or metaphor other underscore the differences between AIDS discourse and reference making life and reinforce AIDS-related messages of distance and danger. Paraphrasing Clatts and Mutchler, all of these terms have the potential for fixing attention on a small range of possible references and direct(ing) attention away from other, equally possible references.

Speakers may not have such outcomes in mind when they use these words and phrases to express references to AIDS. But these are the messages established when speakers use such expressions in text-making, and their use of these expressions coincides with messages about AIDS established by features of sentence syntax, by question-answering strategies, and elements of narrative style which they also employ in those settings. Several features characterize the speakers' use of in this dialogue. First of all, AIDS is, clearly the central in, this discussion, and concerns about AIDS are implicit in of the speakers' statements; however, the term AIDS' never occurs in the respondent's comments.

When references to AIDS are unavoidable, he uses more neutral, highly context dependent synonym; otherwise, he lets the wording of the physician's questions establish the frame of reference for a concise, and usually unelaborated, reply.

Concise, unelaborated responses were especially evident in the opening section of the dialogue. Here the respondent's statements contain noun constructions, but only rarely are they accompanied by verbs.

In other words, he identifies persons or states of activity as appropriate to the discussion, but he leaves the details of the action undescribed.Hence, the respondent notes that his roommate travelled, though he does not explain why he travelled or where he went and denies knowing anything about the roommate's sexual activity while away from home. He indicates that he has friends, though he says nothing about them nor does he explain why, if they are his friends, he has not told them about his illness.

What little lie does say on these themes is presented in sentences dominated by negative markers. The one sentence in this section which does not fit that syntactic pattern contains a single-word, unelaborated comment which serves to bring this line of questioning to a close. Even when the physician's questions probed for greater detail, the respondent's replies continued to be succinct and cryptic, obligating the physician and the linguist to interpret sentence meanings in terms of their own sources of data.

The linkage between the respondent's illness and the roommate's adventurousness while away from home provides the only clue that the living arrangement was personal and intimate, yet that connection has to be inferred from multiple comments of physician and respondent, and is not explicitly indicated in the text on its own.· Respondent comments continued to be tersely constructed during the final section of the interview and, as before, the comments offer only glimpses into the issues under discussion.

This time, however, the glimpses are much more richly detailed, instead of presenting himself as a shadow-figure with only vaguely detailed social connections to those around him, the respondent positions himself as the central actor in the events he identifies. That is, he made the choice to become predominantly homosexual and to be involved in the gay lifestyle. And he was the person eager to explore everything that this lifestyle had to offer. Importantly, the syntax of these comments supports and confirms the messages displayed through the speaker's word choices.

Negative construction, so common to the comments in lines 1-16, do not occur in these statements. Sentence subjects are first person, singular references, and the indicated subject is always the agent, not the recipient, of verb action. The shifts in richness of speaker commentary and assertions of speaker agency' displayed within this text do more than coincide with speaker-controlled changes in text focus. They also show how AIDS-related references to the distant, antisocial other affect the overall form of a speaker's text and influence other areas of his text-based presentation of messages.

In this case, someone who had nothing to say about his own erotic activity when the topic under discussion was HIV illness became quite willing to offer comment on that activity once the topic shifted to a more neutral, less disquieting domain. Initially, other parties the roommate, his unidentified sex partners were the significant actors in the discussion, with the respondent carefully positioning himself at distance from them, from his friends, and from anyone else he had to identify.

Once the topic the importance he assigns to his own actions, compared against the emphasis he placed on the actions of others in that regard. Health educators and policy-makers continue to be perplexed by a contradictory condition widely reported by AIDS researchers and practitioners: gay men will report a high degree of 'correct' risk knowledge but still engage in high-risk erotic activities, all the same.

Stall, Coates, and Hoff found this to be the only common theme in studies of effective AIDS education as of 1988; otherwise, studies to date disagreed quite openly as to factors actually promoting changes in AIDS-related risk behaviour. Reviews of the literature published since that time show that those disagreements have not been resolved. Some researchers, hoping to bring greater clarity to these conditions, have carried out extensive interviews/ discussions with gay men to elicit their rationales for participating in high-risk eroties.

Bolton cautions that comments offered in the objective environment of an interview setting may not coincide with the respondent's actual practice in real-life, erotic domains. Equally serious, researchers elicit first-hand commentary about risky sex but use their own assumptions about erotic risk, rather than clues in the respondents' commentary, to interpret the respondents' explanations for their behaviour. Nearly all of the men offering this excuse felt their behaviour was uncharacteristic of them and attributable to uncontrollable urges, which overwhelmed their intent to use protection. These men typically described these urges as powerful biological needs and drives, which they dubbed passion or 'horniness.'

Gay men who have been sexually active during their gender career will understand the issues which these respondents are describing. In that sense, explaining the appeal of high-risk sex in terms of 'hominess' seems a reasonable research conclusion. But that conclusion ignores other clues to their behaviour which the speakers built into their responses.

Analyzing these statements as texts that is, as products of choice-making, as intended constructions will make those comments more accessible. A described his first encounter with this partner by using which is devoid of agency marking: 'There was unprotected oral sex and unprotected anal sex', Agency can be inferred from his comments, but agency is not formally marked as such description.

The differences in text construction make it necessary to rethink the conclusions which Levine and Siegel drew from these statements. Lust and passion are in these discussion, and they do influence the respondents decisions to participate in high-risk behaviour. However, lust and passion are secondary to the assertions of agency presented in these texts and to effects differences in agency had on decision-making in, each case. Levine and Siegel we correct to their sexual passion as a means of accounting for the participation in unsafe sex.

6

Healthcare of AIDS Patients

In the early stages of HIV illness, palliative treatment can inexpensively relieve some of the pain, discomfort and incontinence that otherwise rob people of the ability to enjoy life and contribute to their family and their community. The opportunistic illnesses that commonly arise early in the course of AIDS can also be treated quite inexpensively. Treatment for thrush, toxoplasmosis and pneumonia/ septicemia can buy one to four years of life at an additional drug cost of $30 to $150—all but the very poor would probably be willing and able to pay for these treatments. Rarer opportunistic illnesses like the fungal diseases tend to occur later in the course of the HIV infection and are more difficult and expensive to treat. Many of the symptoms and opportunistic illnesses that occur in the early stages of AIDS can be effectively treated at low cost.

Unfortunately, the low-cost generic forms of the needed drugs are often unavailable; even when they are available, people often lack information about their efficacy. Governments can address these problems by facilitating the availability of generic drugs needed for palliative care and common opportunistic illnesses. For example, countries with a concentrated or generalised epidemic could add these medications to their list of "essential drugs," which are widely distributed.

Governments can also help patients to make informed decisions by ensuring access to reliable information about the efficacy of various treatment options, both pharmaceuticals and traditional remedies. The degree of government subsidy for treatment will depend on the country's overall health financing policy. The treatments discussed above ease suffering and prolong life but ultimately fail to save the patient's life because none attacks the underlying cause of illness—the continued spread of HIV within the body and the consequent decline of the immune system's ability to recognise and repel biological threats. A few drugs have reduced the levels of HIV in the patient's blood below the ability of laboratory tests to detect it. Unfortunately, these drugs are expensive and complex to administer, their long-term benefits are uncertain and their efficacy varies greatly from one individual to another.

The first drug that showed evidence of inhibiting the spread of the virus in an infected patient was zidovidine (AZT, or ZDV). When AZT was introduced in the late 1980s, the cost of a year's dosage was about $10,000 in industrial countries. By 1997 the cost of a year's dose had fallen to about $2,738 in industrial countries, while Thailand and a few other developing countries had negotiated bulk purchases for as little as $657 per patient per year. However, except for prevention of mother-to-child transmission, AZT rarely provided dramatic benefits, adding perhaps six months of healthy life for the average patient. A more effective therapy involving the use of three antiretrovirals was announced in June 1996. A year later, the U.S. government issued draft guidelines recommending early, aggressive treatment of HIV-infected individuals with triple-drug therapy.

However, it was clear that more time would be needed before the new therapies could be fully assessed. Some individuals taking the medicines in clinical trials have dramatically improved their health and no longer have detectable levels of viral RNA activity. Yet even among these patients, the virus may only be hiding and could re-emerge. And other patients show little or no reduction in viral levels, while still others cannot tolerate the drugs.

As of mid-1997 no studies had yet been completed estimating the average percentage of patients who could benefit from triple-drug therapy or the characteristics of patients most likely to respond favourably—or to relapse. Even if the therapy is shown to be generally effective, three substantial problems will remain: the cost of the drugs themselves, the costs and difficulty of the monitoring needed for the therapy to be effective and problems with patient compliance.

Although all of these problems also exist in industrial countries, they are likely to be especially severe in developing country medical settings. Effective antiretroviral therapy requires a highly trained, specialised physician working in a well-equipped clinic with experience performing a wide range of sophisticated tests and procedures, all of which are in critically short supply in most developing countries. In the event that cost and infrastructure problems could somehow be overcome, patient compliance would continue to pose serious difficulties. Patients undertaking triple-drug therapy must swallow up to 20 pills a day according to a complex schedule related to sleep and meal times.

Failure to follow the schedule increases the chance that the virus will become resistant or that the patient will be too sickened by the drugs to continue treatment. Even well-educated patients with good clinical support have difficulty adhering to this demanding regimen; moreover, patients in the early stages of HIV infection are sometimes not willing to take drugs that make them nauseous when they otherwise feel healthy. In clinical trials in industrial countries, for example, as few as 26 per cent of patients complied with the instructions.

Problems with patient compliance are likely to be worse in low-income countries due to lower education levels and the many other problems that poor people in developing countries face. Even with all these difficulties and uncertainties, many patients in developing countries will ask their physicians for triple-drug therapy, just as patients have attempted to obtain AZT.

Governments will in turn face pressure to buy these drugs and to subsidize the necessary clinical services. When very few people have AIDS, total costs will also be small relative to other government expenditures. Where the AIDS epidemic is severe, health policymakers inside and outside government have sought ways to provide compassionate care at low cost. Three alternatives to expensive inpatient care are outpatient AIDS clinics, hospice care (residential low-technology care for the terminally ill) and home-based care. One innovative program to deliver high-quality treatment of symptoms and opportunistic illnesses without the expense of hospitalisation was an outpatient clinic started in 1989 in Sao Paulo, Brazil. Such clinics are especially well suited to serve urban HIV-positive and AIDS patients who are able to leave their homes. Later in the course of the disease, when the patient is less mobile, the hospice or nursing home provides a lower-cost substitute for inpatient care in a sophisticated referral hospital. However, since such facilities are rarely available in developing countries, the main alternative to the hospital is care at home. Assuming that the average patient with AIDS would survive six months with either type of care, the benefits of home-based care must be measured in reductions of hospitalisation cost: reduced travel time to the hospital for the patient and the patient's caretakers; increased patient satisfaction and comfort; and ancillary benefits to the community, such as improved understanding of the ways to prevent AIDS and decreased stigma toward HIV-positive people.

AIDS will affect the health sector in two ways: by increasing demand and by reducing the supply of a given quality of care at a given price. As a result, some HIV-negative people who would have obtained treatment had there been no epidemic will be unable to do so and total national expenditure on health care will rise, both in absolute terms and as a proportion of national product.

Most people who develop AIDS are prime-age adults. Without AIDS, this 15-to-50 age group accounts for only 10 to 20 per cent of all deaths in a developing country, but these deaths typically generate a disproportionate share of total health care demand. Moreover, since several studies suggest that adults with AIDS use more health care prior to death than those who die of other causes, or even of other prolonged illnesses, the percentage increase in the demand for care by adults is likely to exceed the percentage increase in their mortality due to AIDS. As a result of these two factors, in a country where prime-age adults utilised one-quarter of all health care before AIDS, a given percentage increase in their demand for health care will increase total demand by at least one-quarter of that percentage.

For example, a 40 per cent increase in the mortality rate of prime-age adults will increase total demand by at least 10 per cent, even though total mortality has increased by only 4 per cent to 8 percent. If AIDS patients use expensive antiretroviral therapies, the increase in demand will be much greater. How much the demand for care increases in the aggregate depends on the increase in the prime-age adult death rate, which in turn depends on the level of HIV prevalence and the median time from infection to death.

A stable prevalence rate of 5 per cent among prime-age adults eventually increases their annual mortality by about five deaths per 1,000 adults if the median time from infection to death is ten years, or by about ten deaths if the median time is only five years. A prevalence rate of 30 per cent, such as is observed in Lusaka, Zambia, will increase the number of deaths per 1,000 adults by 30 to 60, depending on the median time to death. In Sub-Saharan Africa, where mortality rates in this age group were as high as five per 1,000 before the epidemic, even a 5 per cent infection rate will double or triple the adult death rate. In a middle-income developing country with adult mortality of one per 1,000, the same endemic level of HIV infection will increase prime-age adult mortality five or tenfold.

Given these parameters, how much will the epidemic increase the demand for care? In a country where adults consume one-quarter of health care prior to the AIDS epidemic, HIV prevalence is constant at 5 per cent of adults; the median time to death is ten years and the baseline mortality rate among prime-age adults is 5 per 1,000, the epidemic will cause a 26 per cent increase in the demand for health care at every price. If the prevalence rate is higher, the median time to death shorter, or the baseline adult mortality rate smaller, percentage increase in demand will be correspondingly greater.Another important factor that may increase demand is insurance. This may take the form of private insurance, a government-run insurance program, or, more typically, health care financed through general taxation. Because a portion of health care costs is often covered by one or more of these types of insurance, the price paid by the patient is usually a fraction of the cost of providing the care. Since insurance enables patients to purchase more care than they would otherwise, it increases the demand for care arising from any given level of illness, thus magnifying the price shock of an AIDS epidemic.

In addition to increasing the demand for care, the AIDS epidemic will reduce the supply available at a given price, in three ways. The magnitude of these effects, discussed below, will generally be larger in the poorest countries with the largest epidemics. The first and largest effect is the increased cost of maintaining a given level of safety for medical procedures. Even without HIV, hospitals and clinics in poor countries may pose a risk to health. Because the AIDS epidemic has greatly increased the risk to patients of existing medical procedures, simply maintaining the level of safety that existed before HIV requires additional hygiene and blood screening, both of which increase the cost of care. In middle to high-income countries, where blood screening and sterilisation of injecting equipment are already the norm, the impact of AIDS is confined to the incremental costs of adding an HIV test to existing tests and using rubber gloves and face masks in situations where they were previously not used. In poor countries, where blood screening and needle sterilisation were lacking before the epidemic, the resources needed to maintain the quality of care in the face of the AIDS epidemic can be substantial.

For example, the annual recurrent budget of the Ugandan Blood Transfusion Service, which was established in response to the epidemic and meets the demands of the entire Ugandan national health care system for clean blood, is estimated to be about $1.2 million, including capital and recurrent costs. This amounts to about 2 per cent of national public health expenditures or about 1 per cent of total national health expenditures. Despite the potentially high costs of blood screening, HIV has greatly increased the justification for a government role in ensuring a safe blood supply. However, there is no convincing rationale for government to subsidize the entire cost of running such a service indefinitely. Blood screening and improved collection procedures will protect blood donors and recipients. However, since average donors and recipients do not engage in unprotected sex with a large number of partners, a person infected while giving or receiving blood is not likely to pass the infection to many others.

Thus, in developing countries where the cost of establishing a safe blood supply is high, blood screening will not be among the more cost-effective approaches to preventing an epidemic based on sexual transmission. To be sure, blood screening and better hygiene will help to prevent the spread of other infectious diseases besides AIDS. Such measures will also reduce the occupational risk of AIDS and other diseases that health care workers face and therefore reduce the amount of additional compensation needed to offset their occupational risk.

Another obvious and politically appealing response to the HIV/AIDS epidemic is to increase the government share of health care costs and thus the overall subsidy for health care. Such a course of action may be especially attractive early in the epidemic, when few people are sick with AIDS. There is an argument for it on economic grounds as well: it would fill the gap created by the failure of the private market to offer health care insurance in poor countries. However, increasing the subsidy to curative care increases the demand for a limited supply. As a result, both effective price and total expenditure will rise by a greater proportion than the increased subsidy alone, or the increased demand arising from the epidemic alone, or even the sum of the two, would suggest.

As more and more people become sick with AIDS, this effect becomes evident in escalating health care expenditures; in a severe epidemic, the burden on the government budget is likely to become unsustainable. To understand how changes in the level of government subsidies affect the impact of the epidemic on the health care sector, we first look at the extent to which governments already subsidize care. Then, taking India as an example, we project the impact of an expanding epidemic at the current subsidy level and an increased subsidy level.

As we shall see, increasing the overall subsidy to care can greatly exacerbate the impact of the epidemic on the health sector.India's government health expenditures grow from$3.2 billion in 1991 to $8 billion in 2010. The second line from the bottom shows the increase in government health spending if India's current steep rise in HIV prevalence continues until 2000, then levels off at a stable 5 per cent. This is about the growth in prevalence seen in countries such as Zambia and Botswana, where focused prevention was not implemented early in the epidemic. The result in India would be to increase the government's expenditure on health in the year 2010 by about one-third, from $8 billion to $10.5 billion. The large expenditure shocks that will result from the AIDS epidemic will create new pressures on health budgets, especially in countries that enter the AIDS epidemic with higher subsidy rates.

Another common health sector response to the HIV/AIDS epidemic is to offer a different subsidy rate depending on whether or not the person receiving care is infected with HIV. Especially in the countries in the nascent stage of the epidemic, HIV-infected people all too frequently experience discrimination, including restricted access to or higher effective prices for health care. As the epidemic advances, however, governments are often pressed to provide special subsidies for the treatment of HIV/AIDS. A bias against those with HIV/AIDS can take many forms, ranging from a singling out of AIDS-specific drug therapies for exclusion from public funding, to outright refusal of service. There are many anecdotes about discrimination against the HIV-infected in health care settings.

In some hospitals, the HIV-infected were placed in special AIDS wards, which were subsequently shunned by fearful health care workers. In others, the HIV-infected were required to pay extra costs for rubber gloves or a private room. In still other cases, the HIV-infected have been denied treatment for common illnesses, perhaps because doctors and nurses mistakenly believed that nothing could be done to help a person with HIV/AIDS. Such discrimination is unfair, unprofessional and unethical. Moreover, it displays ignorance of the many ways, discussed above, in which inexpensive treatments for symptoms and opportunistic illnesses can prolong and improve the lives of people with HIV/AIDS. Government has an important role to play in training medical personnel in order to eradicate all vestiges of discrimination against HIV-infected patients. Yet it is equally unfair and also inefficient, for government to subsidize a higher proportion of the costs of care for patients with HIV than for other patients. Aside from the issue of poverty, there are three ways to justify government subsidies for curative health care:

(1) as an incentive for those with an infectious disease to seek a cure and avoid infecting others,

(2) as health care insurance with universal coverage and mandatory participation through general taxes, or

(3) as government support for a "merit good" or "basic need."

AZT treatment of HIV-infected pregnant women has been shown to reduce transmission at birth, but is still too costly an approach to preventing secondary infections in the poorest countries. With the prominent exception of TB, the treatment of which should be subsidized in all countries, most opportunistic illnesses that afflict the HIV infected are infectious only to other equally sick HIV-infected people.

Governments should avoid two types of health care responses to the epidemic: increasing the overall subsidy to all types of treatment and providing disproportionately large subsidies to treatment of HIV/AIDS. There are nonetheless several ways in which governments can intervene to mitigate the health impact of HIV/AIDS on infected individuals and their families and on the overall health sector.

— Provide information about the efficacy of treatments. Because people with HIV/AIDS are often desperate for treatment and cannot easily research what works, they are especially vulnerable to quackery.

— Subsidise the treatment of infectious opportunistic illnesses and STDs. Subsidised treatment is especially appropriate for tuberculosis, one of the most common opportunistic illnesses to infect AIDS patients, since curing a single case can avert many secondary infections.

— Subsidise the start-up costs for blood safety and AIDS care. The AIDS epidemic has increased the willingness of individuals to pay for certain types of services, such as screening of blood for transfusions and care for the terminally ill. Where these services are lacking, government help with the start-up costs is justified.

— Provide special assistance to the most poor. Countries already make special provision for medical care to the poor. As the AIDS epidemic increases the demand for care, governments may wish to focus such assistance even more on those who can least afford it.

7

Combating AIDS

Absence of a fully developed tradition of theory and method for conducting sex research has restricted the development of new studies, offering AIDS researchers little foundation for the assessment of sexual practices relevant to the spread of HIV, and has limited their ability to contribute significantly to the design of more effective strategies for AIDS prevention. These points are of course hardly novel. On the contrary, many similar concerns have already been raised elsewhere. As the HIV/AIDS epidemic continues to gain force, however, apparently escaping the vast majority of our efforts to contain it as well as the conceptual models that we have constructed in order to understand it, the limitations in our under standing of sexuality and sexual risk in the face of HIV/AIDS nonetheless pose a series of theoretical, methodological, and procedural questions which cannot be Ignored.

Perhaps more than anything else, we are confronted with the urgent need to rethink the models that have guided the dominant response to AIDS thus far. In seeking to review the development of sex research in relation to HIV/AIDS over the course of the past decade, at least two major problems are worth careful consideration:

(1) the fundamental limitations in the dominant theoretical and methodological paradigms that have been used in carrying out research; and

(2) the equally fundamental limitations in the research agenda that has guided the study of sexual behaviour in relation to HIV/AIDS.

These issues are closely interrelated, since the lack of theoretical and methodological development is almost surely linked to the failure to define a more meaningful research agenda, and vice versa. In order to identify some of the problems that they have raised for research or, sexual behaviour in relation to AIDS thus far, as well as to use them as a point departure for thinking about more effective research activities in the future. The lack of preexisting baseline data on human sexuality and, consequently, the urgent need for data collection on behaviours that may be linked to HIV transmission, have of course been widely discussed. Somewhat less attention has been given, however, to the serious limitations; of dominant theoretical and methodological paradigms that have been employed in carrying out such research.

The limitations of such are perhaps most glaring at a theoretical level, as sexual behaviour research within the context of AIDS has almost never been driven by a theory of sexual behaviour. Indeed, in most instances, it has not been driven by any theory at all the emphasis has been on the urgent need for descriptive data apparently based upon the hope that theoretical insights will emerge from such data if we only have enough of it. When, occasionally, a theoretical framework for conceptualizing sexual behaviour has been invoked, it has been at best a minimal one most commonly the conceptualization of sexual desire as a basic human drive, but a drive that is shaped somewhat differently in different social and cultural settings, and that must therefore be described as it manifests itself within these settings. This lack of theoretical development is not, of course, new to AIDS research.

On the contrary, it is, very much, a product result of the particular tradition of sex research that has been incorporated within the field of public health more generally. Emerging, in many ways, as a response to the moral strictures of Victorian society and the science, the primary focus of this tradition has been an attempt to 'demystify' and, in particular, to 'naturalize' human sexual behaviour an attempt to describe, as exhaustively as pos-sible, the forms of sexual expression that exist 'in nature.' The importance of such a perspective should not be underestimated, as it is principally responsible, particularly following the work of Kinsey and his colleagues, for opening up the field of sexual behaviour as an object of scientific investigation rather than as the domain of religion or morality.

At the same time, its legacy, particularly as it has been incorporated into the field of public health, has clearly been problematic a kind of extreme empiricism, which, in the absence of a more convincing theory for the explanation of human sexuality and sexual diversity has focused almost exclusively on documenting behavioural frequencies within a relatively limited range of population groups.

Increasingly, over the course of a number of decades now, work carried out in a variety of disciplines has tended to challenge this naturalist view, focusing instead on what has been described as the 'social and cultural construction' of sexual conduct. In fields such as cultural anthropology, sociology, social psychology, and history, attention has increasingly focused on the social, cultural, economic, and political forces shaping sexual behaviour in different settings, together with the complicated meanings associated with sexual experience on the part of both individuals and social groups. For the most part, however, the impact of such developments has been extremely limited, particularly within the context of public health and the health sciences, and a more naturalist approach, in spite of its theoretical limitations, has largely continued to dominate the discussion of sexual behaviour and sexual health. The result of this general lack of theoretical development has been a relative poverty in the conceptual frameworks of much sexual behaviour research in relation to HIV /AIDS.

Sexual desire has been treated, in many ways, as a kind of given, and the social and cultural factors shaping sexual experience in different settings have largely been ignored, even when lip service has been paid to their potential importance. In keeping with the dominant tendencies' in much health behaviour research, has been placed largely on the individual determinants of sexual behaviour and behaviour change, and the diverse social, cultural, economic, and political factors potentially influencing or even shaping sexual experience have more often than not been ignored.

A range of theoretical perspectives based on quite distinct premises have been largely absent from the field of AIDS research, mid the various insights that such perspectives might potentially offer have rarely been incorporated in AIDS research findings. A series of methodological limitations can be associated, in large part, with the theoretical limitations described above again seriously inhibiting the quality of the sexual behaviour research that has been carried out in response to AIDS.

Throughout this period, the dominant focus has been on the use of survey research methods, and the key question addressed in the design of research has almost inevitably been how to make these methods more effective in the different contexts in which AIDS research must be carried out in developing countries, for example, or among problematically defined target populations such as homosexual men or intravenous drug users and so on. Such an approach has fit reasonably well within the framework of a research agenda defined in terms of epidemiological questions, for example, or of psychological models of behavioural change.

Counting the frequency of sexual acts, if carried out effectively, can clearly offer important insights concerning the course of the HIV/AIDS epidemic in specific settings. In much the depending upon one's assumptions, measuring psychosocial indicators may offer in sight into the propensity for risk reduction. The subjective and inter-subjective meanings associated with it may be far more important. The social construction of sexual excitement and desire, ways in which sexual identities are formed and transformed, the relations of power and domination that may shape and structure sexual interactions, and the social/ sexual networks that channel and condition the selection of potential sexual partners may all be salient issues that must be taken into account in developing more effective strategies for AIDS prevention.

Yet, to the extent that sexual behaviour research in relation to AIDS has largely closed itself off from a wider range of theoretical frameworks, it has also closed itself off, at least in part, from any number of potentially important methodological approaches that might well lead to new, and perhaps quite different, insights about such issues approaches such as ethnographic description, linguistic analysis, and so on. The lack of theoretical and methodological development characterizing much of the sexual behaviour research carried out during the course of the first decade of the AIDS epidemic has also clearly been exaggerated or aggravated by the absence of more systematic planning and the failure to articulate a coherent research agenda capable of directing or guiding long-term research activities within an inter national or global framework.

We have been unable to define and implement a more comprehensive research agenda on the full range of sexual behaviour and sexual diversity that might truly be capable of guiding epidemiological insights rather than simply following upon their heels. In the absence of such an agenda, changing demands on the part of policy makers, and often funding agencies as well, have tended to shift more rapidly than behavioural research on sexuality can accompany. An early emphasis on descriptive research has thus given way, increasingly, to a focus on intervention research.

Research attention to certain behavioural groups has given way to a focus on others again, sometimes for good reason. And so on. Yet such changes have taken place without the benefit of any kind of wider framework or vision concerning the long-term research issues that must be addressed in the study of sexual behaviour. Changes of direction are of course expected in the development of behavioural research in any area. In the case of research on sexual behaviour within the context of the international AIDS pandemic, however, the lack of a wider research, agenda developed on a global level has all too often led to the lack of sustained research development to the abandonment of work that has only just begun, or the inability to implement studies that fail fit the model of this year's fashions. Only a few years ago, it was virtually impossible to find funding for studies of women's sexual behaviour in relation to HIV/AIDS. Today, it is equally or more difficult to find funds for studies of homosexuality.

The limitations implicit in such short-sighted visions are all too evident, and pose a serious threat to our ability to develop a longer-term understanding of the international AIDS pandemic. Globally, in a world in which research priorities are often established far from the sites where research must actually be carried out, the results of such disparities can be a fundamental distortion of reality. Just one example here might be the way in which reported changes in gay an behaviour in San Francisco or Amsterdam have sometimes been used to suggest that it is unnecessary to investigate questions of same-sex behaviour change in Rio de Janeiro, Bangkok, Mexico City Lagos, and so on. Ultimately the, together with the limitation of existing theoretical and methodological models for the study of sexual behaviour in relation to HIV/AIDS, the lack of a meaningful research agenda has made it almost impossible to elaborate a set of coherent and consistent research priorities.

Throughout the course of the past decade, sexual behaviour research in response to AIDS has thus been faced with the peculiarly intense pressure of rapidly changing priorities an almost constant sense of putting out fires in which sexual behaviour research activities have consistently lagged behind the identification of epidemiological 'hot spots.' In seeking to respond to key issues being raised by the epidemiology of AIDS, early studies of gay and bisexual behaviour were initiated very quickly. Later, as our understanding of the potential shape and size of the epidemic began to change, so too did our understanding of the topical areas that must be addressed studies of heterosexual behaviour in the general population, of women's sexual practices, and so on, have gradually followed.

In general, however, AIDS case reporting and, to a lesser extent, seroprevalence rates, combined with our own sometimes distorted perceptions of these issues, have tended to define priorities and sexual behaviour research, with few exceptions, has tended to offer little guidance in pointing the direction for epidemiological inquiry. It is perhaps especially worth noting that one of the very few exceptions to the general rule would seem to be the record of ethnographic work carried out over the course, of the past decade in response to AIDS. It is symptomatic that ethnographic studies of sexual meanings have been fundamental in calling into question the hegemony of epidemiological categories the relevance, not only for prevention but even for epidemiological purposes, of groups such as men who have sex with men, female 'commercial sex workers, or the female partners of male injecting drug users.

Ethnographic research, preoccupied with the nuances of local knowledge, the social and cultural particularities of sexual experience and he complex networks of power that condition not only the spread of HIV but the ways in which social systems respond to AIDS has in fact developed one of the few bodies of knowledge that would appear to offer insights that might meaningfully guide epidemiological inquiry in different settings rather than simply being carried in its wake. Even if ethnographic studies and cross-cultural analysis have shown promise in opening up new understandings, particularly in relation to sexuality and HIV/AIDS, such approaches have received relatively little attention or support as part of a broader, institutionalized research response to the international AIDS pandemic.

The international research agenda, even in the social sciences, has continued to be largely overdetermined by epidemiological concerns, a id the potential insights of other approaches, based on theoretical foundations, have been largely ignored. And, in much the same way that the biomedical establishment has continued to define the kinds of approaches that will dominate the research agenda in relation to sexuality, the complex relationship between knowledge and power in the field of AIDS has been all the more problematic within an international framework. It is by now abundantly clear that available resources for research on HIV and AIDS generally in the developing world add up to but a fraction of the resources available for such work in the industrialized West, and this is clearly all the more true in relation to social and behavioural research in particular.

The constantly changing, sometimes contradictory, priorities concerning what are considered to be relevant research topics would seem to be especially pronounced in the definition of an international research agenda in relation to sexuality and sexual behaviour. In spite of the obvious epidemiological importance of increased understanding concerning sexual behaviour in some regions of the developing world for a variety of factors which, depending oil the setting, have ranged from a lack of local research capacity to moral political reservation on the part of local authorities or to a lack of have combined to limit sexual be research primarily a to developed countries.

While a number of initiatives have been planned to respond to, diverse circumstances and rapid changes in policy and personnel have meant that relatively little has actually been done. And even where work has been initiated, the tendency has often been to simply apply the dominant research methodologies developed for the study of sexual behaviour in the quite different research settings found in many developed nations. Even though the application of survey research methods has often proven problematic, as well as expensive and slow to implement, for example, there has been very little attempt to respond to these limitations through methodological innovation to develop research methodologies and research agendas that will be better suited to the actual research conditions and Priorities that in fact exist at a global level.

It was in 1984 that the Philippine government first confirmed a clinical case of AIDS in the country. As in many developing countries, the initial public response was one of indifference, with the problem perceived as a 'foreign disease' and, later, as a 'sex worker disease.' Such perce-ptions were reinforced by the demographic pattern of initial reports, with most of the identified HIV positive cases involving women sex workers servicing US military bases in the country.

Starting in 1988, the Philippine government, mainly through foreign grants, to intensify its HIV prevention activities through information, education and communication (IEC) campaigns. The result has been a number of research projects conducted mainly in order to support the IEC campaigns.

This chapter will concentrate on some of the operational research activities. Specificallythe projects in Metro Manila. They are

1) The knowledge, attitudes, and practices (KAP) survey conducted by a private market research firm in 1989 in Metro Manila among 'sentinel groups' with a total of 900 respondents, the results if which we are contracted to analyse and synthesize in 1990-1991.

2) An IEC project for medical and nursing students that included a survey of 960 students in Metro

Manila universities, implemented by the Health Action Information Network (HAIN);

3) An IEC project for male sex workers, implemented by HAIN; and

4) An ongoing IEC project for men who have sex with men, implemented by The Library Foundation.

The interest is, in turn, based on my teaching courses on Sex and Culture and on Medical Anthropology at the University of the Philippines and on my work with HAIN, a non governmental organization servicing community-based health programmes. As with other social scientists in developing countries, we felt that the problem of AIDS had raised the challenge of bringing back into public discourse frank and open discussion of sexuality and gender issues.

The Philippines went through periods of colonization under Spain and the United States, often described in the media as 300 years of the convent followed by 50 years of Hollywood. The description can be misleading, implying two different and discrete sociocultural 'waves' crashing on procolonial culture and eventually creating a homogenous 'Filipino culture.'

The Spaniards did introduce their strongly patriarchal and erotophobic brand of Roman Catholicism, but this found continuity with the fire-and-brimstone moralism of American Protestant evangelicals.

The US colonial period also introduced secular—often medical explanatory models that could coexist with or even reinforce religious paradigms, e.g., the labelling of homosexuality as a disease or the use of Freudian explanations to explain sexual orientation. A positivist tradition in social research, established during the US colonial period, tends to limit analysis to superficial expressions of sexual and political cultures without adequately addressing the dynamics of these cultures, including the interaction between religious and secular sexual ideologies, or between dominant and popular cultures. There is, for instance, the frequently cited work of the Jesuit psychologist Bulatao, who described 'split-level Christianity' sharp differences between expressed norms and actual behaviour and attributed this to the coexistence of 'Christian' and 'pagan' theological systems in the Philippines. Bulatao's work includes examples of sexual behaviour. His article calls for an individual change of values as the solution.

It is not surprising that with the spread of HIV and AIDS, such forms of moralistic analysis have once again emerged, often creating common ground for conservatives and progressive who target moral decadence' as the cause of HIV. The lack of a critical tradition in research into sexuality can be serious.

When we began the HIV prevention programmes, one of our major problems was the lack of published studies on sexuality in the Philippines. In fact, the only noteworthy publications on general issues surrounding sexuality the Philippines have been produced only in the last two years, consisting of three books by a Filipino clinical psychologist and sex therapist, Margarita Go-Singco Holmes.

Another reflection of the lack scholarly research is the fact that there are only publications, now both quite dated, that are worth citing for Filipino men who have with men,' one by the late anthropologist Donn Hart and other a four country study by Whitam and Robin Mathy, both articles concentrating on transvestite cultures. As the HIV/AIDS problem grows in the Philippines, the urgency for action-oriented research has become even more pressing, but HIV prevention and control programmes will remain off-course as social scientists and programme implementors fail to recognize their own cultural blind spots.

These contradictions are found even among people involved in HIV/AIDS work and are best exemplified by Poisoned Blood, a film documentary produced by a Filipino AIDS activist in which AIDS is depicted as a product of the moralism of Roman Catholicism; the US colonizers' 'sexual permissiveness'; the US military bases in the Philippines; the non-illegal status of homosexuality; and the Marcos dictatorship's promotion of sexual tourism. Much of the literature on sex and culture has focused on debates between social constructivists and essentialists.

A provocative article by Vance, dealing with anthropology and the study of sexuality suggests that the debate has little impact on many anthropologists. Vance argues that the research has in fact been dominated by what she calls the 'cultural influence model', one that recognizes the role of society and culture in shaping sexual behaviour and attitudes but which continues to accept, as a given, a universal and biologically determined 'bedrock of sexuality.' The lack of theoretical discussion, particularly for a developing country such as the Philippines where he need for such debates has been pushed aside because of the dominance of biomedical researchers, who use social scientists simply to gather 'baseline data.'

The absence of debates on theories and models raises serious questions about the validity of the social and behavioural research being conducted, since such research, in the absence of theoretical grounding, is more vulnerable to reducing sexuality to 'quantifiable' behaviour number of times for particular forms of sexual activity divorced from its sociocultural context.

Even attempts to recognize the sociocultural context of sexuality id to adopt some form of cultural relativism, are inadequate when comes to dealing with realities, and use this term in the sense of hat is 'real' subjectively for the individual, as well as what is 'real' objectively, for an outside observer. Let us take the phrase 'men who have sex with men,' abbreviated as 'MSM' now widely used in HIV/AIDS programmes. The phrase was introduced, apparently by Western researchers, in an attempt to introduce neutral language as opposed to what was construed to be Western constructs: 'gay' or even 'homosexual, it is difficult to produce a more appropriate phrase than 'men who have sex with men,' but the label is very much behaviourally fixated, precluding identity and, more importantly, gender.

The useage of the term MSM has produced some rather positive and intriguing results. Men who have sex with men' is also a 'Western' term that emerged, consciously or not, out of an essentialist perspective and that IEC campaigns integrating this term into a plan of action could restrict the potentials of such projects to reach this population, mainly because it shunts off cultural contexts that are important in understanding behaviour. In the Philippines, for instance, the term 'gay' has been incorporated into daily discourse and although it has different uses in different settings, the term does carry meaning, including a sense of sexual and social identity for many Filipinos.

The Library Foundation's HIV prevention workshops for 'men who have sex with men.' Organizers faced a minor crisis when they had an applicant who self-identified as being 'a gay' but had no sexual experience, either with other men or with women. He was allowed to join the workshop. One organizer explained, 'He's a gay. He's an MSM.' It was an extraordinary instance of an academic, behaviourally oriented term—men who have sex with men— being appropriated, and transformed, into a social marker. The issue here goes beyond semantics, The danger lies in the use of behaviour as a starting point, and ending there.

If social science research dissociates itself from sociocultural contexts, explanations for behaviour will be greatly weakened. Already, we find many examples of HIV social science to inputs that reflect behaviourist psychology again. Thus, many research projects concentrate on health psychologists' behavioural change models, resulting in an often futile search for 'psychographic' traits that facilitate or hinder the initiation and maintenance of behavioural change.

Unfortunately, the cross-cultural validity of 'locus of control'—as a construct and as a variable—remains dubious. Yet, so much of the research in HIV/AIDS projects in the Philippines— following US models— attempts to measure this locus of control and its correlations with behavioural change for HIV risk reduction. Not surprisingly, this correlation could not be established in the Philippine studies, since Rotter's model, as applied, fails to consider many significant macrovariables that shape, as well as determine, this locus of control.

In retrospect, this should have been anticipated, since the concept of internal locus of control, presumed to be one of, if not the most important determinants of behavioural change, fails to consider the possibility that there may in fact be a collective locus of control that is neither externally nor internally oriented. Support for HIV/AIDS research, specifically into the social and behavioural aspects, has often been in the form of one-year grants where the research component is meant to support IEC activities.

By necessity the research has to be much like orthodox sex: short, quick, almost mechanical. More disturbing was the fact that the statements had been translated with a lack of linguistic equivalence and, more importantly, conceptual equivalence and cultural appropriateness. The problems in translation lead us back to problems in the theoretical framework, i.e., an assumption that behaviour, and its 'determinants, 'can be easily transformed into measurable variables without due consideration for the subtle texture of culture. We will cite two examples here.

First, a statement lifted from Rotter's I-E Scale for locus of control—we have often found that what is going to happen will happen'—was totally distorted in its translation into Filipino, being transformed into the statement that: 'Usually, what one expects to happen will happen.'

Second, a statement—We are aggressive'—was used as a measure for 'individualism,' which was in turn presumed to be in direct opposition to 'conformity.'

The underlying assumption was that 'individualism' presented a better prognosis for the chances of behavioural change, an assumption that is, of course, controversial. The problem here is complex because the statement is itself culturally inappropriate. Cross-cultural differences create other problems, not just in translation. In many other surveys conducted in conjunction planning IEC materials.

Likert scales are almost always used. Yet my experience, with surveys in the Philippines is that 'strong agree' is a distinction of minimum value. In the words a peasant health worker, the agree or you don't. There is no 'somewhat.' Yet survey after in HIV projects insist on using such scales.

Because of this HAIN's surveys now use agree, disagree or don't know/not sure, which incidentally, does make data processing simpler and more rapid, if this is the objective. For instance, among medical and nursing students, we encountered what seemed to be a contradiction in attitudes toward homosexuality. In our self administered questionnaires used by the students, 27.4 per cent agreed with the statement 'Homosexuality is a disease' and 86.4 per cent agreed with the statement 'It is a sin to have sex with another person of the same sex.' At the same time, 47.6 per cent of the respondents felt that 'Homosexuality is merely a different kind of life-style.'

The inclusion of three different questions in the survey itself, supplemented by focus group discussions, showed that the figures were not necessarily contradictory; in fact, it showed how the medical and nursing students compartmentalize their attitudes to ward homosexuals and homosexuality.

Moral statements elicited more rigid responses while a secular label, 'disease,' tended to be used less often. Straddling religious and medical stigmatization was the statement on 'different kind of life-style,' a neutral area where some degree of tolerance could be expressed.

Whether these views reflect homophobia, and how they may affect the medical and nursing students' willingness to work with homosexuals, would of course be separate issues that need other research methodologies to complement the survey findings. There are rapid qualitative methods that can be used, but they do tend to take more time, and this seems to discourage social and behavioural scientists from utilizing them, despite the fact that such methods, including focus group discussions, can generate vital information. Another example comes from our work with medical and nursing students, where we persistently found agreement with the statement that: 'People with AIDS should be isolated.' We found this important enough to feed back to the students in a final consultative workshop. The explanation was simple: one student said that among medical and nursing students, the concept of 'isolation' does not mean discrimination against people with AIDS (PWAs), since 'isolation' here could have meant protecting PWAs from opportunistic infections, rather than protecting society from the PWAs.

The logic is clear, and it certainly is not limited to Filipino medical and nursing students. For anthropologists, it is important that we recognize the cultures' from which people come, including the 'biomedical' culture that plays such a dominant role today. The rich texture of culture is all too often sacrificed in surveys. Often, it is not the survey itself that may be flawed, but research design that reflects disembodied empiricism and noncritical adoption of research instruments.

Gujarat AIDS Prevention Unit

The goals of the Gujarat AIDS Prevention Unit are as follows:

— To help ensure safe blood supply to the people.

— To protect commercial blood donors from HIV infection through unsterile equipment and procedures at the blood collection centres, and through other risk behaviours such as unprotected sexual intercourse.

— To protect the personnel working in blood collection centres from accidental infection with HIV in the course of their work.

To achieve these objectives the unit developed the following action plan:

— Educate commercial blood donors about safe blood-giving and how to practice safer sex.

— Test commercial blood donors for HIV infection, accompanied by pre- and post-test counselling.

— Provide commercial blood donors with alternative income-generating opportunities.

— Upgrade the existing guidelines for the prevention of infection and for handling body fluids in commercial blood collecting centres.

— Educate the staff at blood collection centres about the possibility of accidental transmission of HIV.

The achievements of the Gujarat AIDS Prevention Unit are encouraging and significant, even if modest in the national context. The unit now have plans to help people who sell their blood for a living by providing them with vocational training and alternative income-generating activities.

The unit also plan to establish, together with the commercial blood donors themselves, a co-operative blood banking system through which blood could be collected from people irrespective of their HIV status. This blood could then be screened and seropositive samples could be sold to research organisations involved in developing vaccines.

The HIV-free blood would be sold to pharmaceutical laboratories. The project has helped to ensure a safe blood supply for the people of Ahmedabad, as well as helping to protect people involved in the blood collection industry from HIV infection.

AIDS Prevention Programmmes in Tamil Nadu

During October 1988, the PANOS Institute, U.K. commissioned Shyamla Nataraj, at that time a Madras-based fireelance journalist with little interest in or knowledge of AIDS, to write about a group of 30 women sex workers who had been diagnosed HIV-positive and were being detained by the police in Madras.

Because of official fears of publicity, it took Shyamla six months to gain access to the women, and when eventually she did, it was a very emotional and shocking experience. Unable to drop the matter after writing her article, she sought legal advice and decided to take the Government of the State of Tamil Nadu to court for unlawful detention of the women. Shyamla eventually won the case and the women were released in July 1990. While the court case was still being contested, however, Shyamla had been travelling around South India to investigate what support services were available for people with HIV/AIDS, but had found none at all. She became increasingly worried about what would happen to the women if and when they were finally released from detention.

Legal action alone, she realized, was of little use without a supportive social infrastructure. She was also struck by the almost complete lack of AIDS awareness at all levels of society, including among NGOs and community groups. Upon returning to Madras she established a link with the Voluntary Health Services Centre in Madras, who agreed to provide her with a bank account for channelling funds and to rent her an office.

After several anxious months the project finally received financial assistance from the WHO Partnership Programme (in collaboration with the

PANOS Institute) and the Ford Foundation. Shyamla had begun linking up with existing NGO networks in South India, especially those of the Voluntary Health Association, the Association of Voluntary Agencies and the Social Welfare Board of Tamil Nadu State.

In February 1991 she organized the first one-day, district-level workshop for NGOs in the Tirunelveli District Tamil Nadu. By September 1991, while still awaiting funding, she had organized twelve district-level workshops, with more than 200 NGOs participating. She had also developed a calendar and booklets, in English and Tamil, containing basic information about AIDS, and distributed copies of these to the NGOs participating in the workshops.

For most participants these workshops were the first time they had ever received any information about AIDS, apart from occasional stories in the mass media. They reported that the experience helped them to clear up their misconceptions and fill important gaps in their knowledge. In March 1992 SIAAP organized a five-day training workshop for 60 representatives of 45 NGOs from all over the State of Tamil Nadu.

The topics covered included in-depth HIV/AIDS information, communication skills and funding. The participants also explored ways of networking more effectively among NGOs doing AIDS-related work in South India. The workshops so far organized have shown that NGOs, however well-motivated, need considerable help in planning AIDS intervention programmes. The NGOs that have participated in the workshops come from a wide range of ideological backgrounds and have different organizational capacities. Some are very cautious about becoming involved in new, potentially sensitive or controversial issues—such as HIV and AIDS —outside their existing areas of activity.

Most NGOs agreed that sexually transmitted diseases (STDs) were a common problem in their communities, but they felt unable to talk openly about the topic, or to provide diagnostic and clinical services to those affected, or even to forge links with organizations providing such services. Condom promotion was rare: most NGOs involved in health care concentrated on family planning methods which required women to take responsibility for contraception. Few NGOs had much experience of collecting and analysing information to enable them to assess their programme needs. Many had difficulty in identifying possible intervention strategies for STD/HIV, control and prevention, tending to stick to approaches with which they were already familiar. Programme monitoring and evaluation were almost nonexistent.

Most importantly, NGO staff were unaccustomed to talking with their clients about sex and sexuality, and needed help in developing communication skills in this area. SIAAP received its first opportunity to provide follow-up support to an NGO when, in April 1991, the Madras Christian Council of Social Services (MCCSS) asked for help in setting up an AIDS education programme in some of the slums where they had been working.

SIAAP helped MCCSS to design and conduct a survey to assess the needs of the slum communities, to develop an appropriate intervention strategy and programmed, and to recruit and train staff. It soon became clear that in order to integrate the AIDS programme into the work of the organization, all the MCCSS staff needed information and training on HIV/AIDS.

SIAAP worked with MCCSS staff to help them' overcome their reluctance to talk about sex and to encourage non-judgemental attitudes. The work with MCCSS was very valuable for SIAAP's own staff as well, giving them the chance to actually experience what they were suggesting other NGOs should do. In August 1991 SIAAP appointed G. Kumaresan (Kumar) to plan and implement a project aiming to protect long-distance lorry drivers and their sexual partners against HIV infection and other STDs.

As in many other parts of the world, long-distance lorry drivers in South India are a group at high risk of contracting HIV infection and other STDs.

Spending most of their working life on the road, away from their families, most drivers regularly engage in sex with partners other than their wives. Kumar brought with him two years experience of an HIV/STD prevention programme in Madras. Originally the programme had tried distributing condoms to female prostitutes, but it soon became clear that the women were in no position to insist on their use.

A more effective strategy was to concentrate on the prostitutes' clients. Shifting the responsibility to the clients also avoided the implication— too often conveyed— that prostitutes are uniquely responsible for spreading HIV and other STDs, and that their clients are merely victims.

Kumar began the SIAAP initiative in October-November 1991 with a survey of long-distance lorry drivers who passed through Puzhal checkpoint. The survey found that over 1,000 drivers and cab assistants passed through the checkpoint every day. Interviews with 200 drivers found that almost 90 per cent visited prostitutes but few used condoms. More than 90 per cent had suffered from an STD, and all were keen to learn how to avoid contracting STDs, including AIDS, in future. SIAAP opened its health education booth at Puzhal in January 1992. A health educator meets with drivers individually in the booth to talk about HIV and AIDS and other sexually transmitted diseases. He also provides at least ten drivers a day with a pack of five condoms, after demonstrating their correct use on a model of a penis. Group discussions are also held. These always elicit a few laughs and help to bring down barriers against condom use. Once a week a video is also shown, mixing AIDS information with entertainment. The booth is well accepted because it focuses on something its clients really want: prevention and treatment of STDs. Condoms are promoted not only for the prevention of AIDS and other STDs, but also as a family planning device.

Kumar believes that about 75 per cent of condoms distributed are used for the purpose intended —most of the remainder are used for more ingenious purposes such as stopping oil leaks in lorry engines. In April 1992, for the first time, the booth advertised that a medical team would come one evening and carry out STD testing. Over 30 customers turned up. Those with positive results were informed on their next stop, and sent for treatment at a clinic in the city. Since approximately the same population of drivers uses this route, over time the results of STD testing will give a reliable indication of the impact of the programme. The possibility of offering HIV testing is still under consideration—so far only one driver has expressed an interest in being tested.

The SIAAP health education booth, in itself, will have only a small impact on the spread of HIV and AIDS in South India. Its importance is that it represents a new strategy of AIDS control and prevention in South India, based on an acceptable approach to an occupational group at high risk of contracting the disease. The project has yet to create sufficient demand for condoms to sell them at cost, but it has developed an approach that can be replicated by other organizations on other trucking routes, at bus stations, in ports, and wherever the long-distance lifestyle encourages sexual straying.

Already five NGOs have asked SIAAP to help them set up similar projects in other parts of South India. Virtually no HIV/AIDS intervention programmes for women, as a group, in India. The few programmes that do exist are targeted specifically at women engaged in prostitution. The women tend to be regarded, however, as pools of infection rather than as human beings with their own problems, needs and rights. The emphasis is usually on containing the spread of HIV infection into the community, rather than on providing care, support services and information to the women concerned. Recognizing the basic injustice and practical inadequacy of such an approach, SIAAP has started working with some of the women engaged in prostitution in the city of Madras.

In a conscious effort to move away from the usual stereotyped approach to sex workers, SIAAP tries to put the women themselves at the centre of the programme. SIAAP was aware that women sex workers viewed their own health as only one concern amongst many. Their main felt needs were for security in the face of the oppressive legal and social system within which they operate, and facilities for the care and education of their children. SIAAP therefore decided to address these two felt needs alongside specifically health-related issues. In the next phase of the project, SIAAP plans to make counselling and STD services available as well. SIAAP also plans to arrange for school sponsorship for the women's children.

SIAAP is working with a group of women activists and lawyers to examine ways of removing or restructuring the existing laws on prostitution, so that the women are not at the mercy of the entrenched, male-dominated control structure. SIAAP established a volunteer training programme in order to help equip people with the knowledge, skills and self-confidence they need to communicate with their peers about HIV and AIDS, in December 1991. By April 1992 three training workshops had been run for 25 volunteers. The first group consisted mainly of students, but subsequent groups have included a wider cross-section of the population first on basic information about HIV/AIDS, then moving on to more complex issues, and finally onto means of communicating about AIDS.

The potential of various means of communication is explored—posters, videos, oral presentations, discussions, one-to-one interactions, skits and street plays. Participants are encouraged to think about what forms of communication are most appropriate for their own peer education activities. Although the feedback so far has been very encouraging, the programme does not take place on a regular basis. Training sessions are organized only in response to specific requests from potential volunteers. Working in the slums of Madras brought home to SIAAP staff the need for STD services as well as AIDS education.

The presence of an STD greatly increases the chances of HIV transmission between sexual partners. Without effective STD services, AIDS education in itself can have only limited value. SIAAP therefore believes that the diagnosis and treatment of STDs should be a key part of any strategy of AIDS control and prevention. Yet there was very little reliable information about the actual prevalence of STDs and the diagnostic and treatment services available. SIAAP therefore engaged Dr. Roman Solomon to carry out a study to provide this information.

The study found that men were generally well aware of the dangers of STDs and sought medical attention (including penicillin injections) after risky sex. Women, however, went for treatment of STDs only if they had a visible problem, and then almost invariably to private practitioners. Very few women sought treatment for STDs at government hospitals and health centres, due to the lack of female STD specialists, the absence of privacy, the judgemental attitudes of doctors, the scarcity of specialist STD clinics and the cost of travelling to the few clinics available.

NGOs working in the slum areas tended to concentrate on basic MCH services, referring STD cases to the general hospital. The study identified the urgent need for STD diagnostic and treatment services to be provided in the slums, preferably by a mobile clinic capable of covering a larger population than one located in a hospital or health centre. SIAAP is currently exploring ways of trying to meet this need. The scope and volume of SIAAP's work have increased dramatically since its humble beginnings, in January 1991, as a project with a one-year time span. Now it is registered as a Trust—a fully fledged NGO with the right to apply for and receive funds directly.

SIAAP now has three main roles. First, it functions as a resource centre, helping NGOs to integrate HIV/AIDS prevention and control into existing community development programmes by providing informa-tion, training, technical support and materials. Second, it facilitates networking among NGOs in South India so that they can learn from one anothers' experiences and also assist one another in various ways. And third, it implements its own community-based activities: the projects for lorry drivers and women in prostitution, soon to be followed by the telephone information service and the drop-in centre. The pressure to expand in order to provide urgently needed services also has financial implications.

SIAAP's initial funding has been from foreign donors. The staff and members of the SIAAP Trust would prefer the programme's activities to be funded entirely from local sources—including government agencies, charitable organizations, the private business sector, individual donors and community groups. They recognize, however, that this ideal may not be attainable in the near future. It is unlikely that the AIDS epidemic will wait for self-sustaining development to be achieved.

Although some of SIAAP's future activities may well be funded by local donors, others will probably still be dependent on external support. In the space of less than two years, SIAAP has helped to give NGOs in South India a headstart in planning AIDS control and prevention programmes that are integrated into existing community development activities.

8

Psychiatric Treatments for AIDS

Psychiatric facilitation of primary care for HIV patients may affect survival, given the association between survival and lack of medical care, higher T-helper, also known as CD_4, cell count at the initial visit, and pneumocystis carinii pneumonia prophylaxis and antiretroviral therapy.

Consult/liaison psychiatry for AIDS

Consult/liaison psychiatry is a speciality area within the area of psychiatry. This function provides a remarkable opportunity to influence patient care without being directly responsible for the patient. This unique perspective often results in a more neutral evaluation than is given by primary-care providers, nursing staff, and social workers who have ongoing interactions with the patient and who may be emotionally involved. One assumption in having psychiatrists service as consultants is that direct-care providers recognize the need for psychiatric consultation. This is a documented problem throughout medicine and is not unique to HIV/AIDS.

Psychiatric liaison services tend to work toward better recognition of psychiatric illness in primary-care settings, as well as assist in the discussion of various legal and ethical issues confronted in the care of complicated patients.

Liaisons take a more proactive role: affiliating with specific providers or clinics, providing continual reinforcement regarding the importance of psychiatric intervention, and bridging gaps between more medically oriented providers and psychosocial or spiritual heaters. The psychiatric consultant/liaison relies heavily on the relationships forged with direct-care providers. Without the information obtained from discussion with these providers or from review of their chart notes, the psychiatric consultant cannot complete his/her assessment. Without support from the staff caring directly for the patient, the best-formed treatment plan will surely fail. One key outcome of having psychiatrists serve as educators is the reduction of stigma associated with mental illness. HIV/AIDS is a disease already characterized by shame, discrimination, and misunderstanding.

When psychiatric illness is added to this tenuous situation, even the most empathic caregiver can succumb to stereotypes and frustration. Psychiatrists, because of their unique biological perspective, can assist HIV/AIDS providers to recognize better psychiatric illness and understand better psychiatric pharmacological subtleties. Psychiatrists can educate other physicians, physician assistants, and nurse practitioners in prevention of iatrogenic disease due to medication toxicity. Psychiatrists, because of their appreciation for the psychosocial/spiritual characteristics of the patient, can listen carefully to providers' and family members' concerns, presenting their information in a manner that the recipient can relate directly to the patient or loved one.

Optimal care for HIV/AIDS patients requires an educational component for patients, providers, and family members.

Psychiatry is not synonymous with psychotherapy. In fact, in recent years some psychiatrists have distanced themselves from the practice of psychotherapy and embraced the definition of psychiatry as strictly a medical discipline. Nevertheless, 50 per cent of residents in psychiatric training are in therapy and believe that therapy is essential to becoming a psychiatrist.

The "art" of medicine resides in the understanding and expertise that addresses that which is human, such as relationships, conscious and unconscious thought, and the complexity of cc volitional" behaviour.

Psychiatry, and medicine in general, would suffer tremen-dously if no medical discipline devoted its time and resources to the better understanding and practice of this art. Concerns regarding cost of care and limited funding may preclude psychiatrists from only performing psychotherapy in the future.

Psychiatric psychotherapy may one day be restricted to complicated patients with severe personality disorders or who require both medications and psycho-therapy. Because of their ability to integrate medical and psychosocial/spiritual perspectives, psychiatrists treating HIV/AIDS patients may be in a unique position to differentiate neurologic sequelae of the virus, psychiatric illness needing medications, psychological distress, and existential dilemmas.

The word psychiatry stems from the Greek for mind and soul; psychiatrists are healers of the mind and the soul. Advances in the late 20th century established a union among the mind, the soul, and the brain that should not end in divorce. Psychiatrists must work diligently to strengthen this union if HIV/AIDS patients are to be served properly. The changing demographics of the HIV/AIDS population suggest an increasing need for psychiatric services in the 21st century. As patients continue to live longer with the disease, there will be a greater opportunity for development of psychiatric illness, both as a result of HIV neurological disorders and as a reaction to living with a chronic illness. It is hoped that efforts to strengthen the collaborative partnerships among primary-care providers, non-physician providers of mental health services, and psychiatrists will lead to increased recognition of psychiatric morbidity in HIV/AIDS patients, for diagnosis always precedes proper treatment.

The epidemic's movement into populations with multiple problems increases the complexity of addressing psychiatric illness in HIV/AIDS patients. Psychiatrists wishing to work with HIV/AIDS patients must prepare to leave the private practice and medical clinic settings in which they currently work. Creative treatment approaches, including housing programs for people with mental illness, substance use, and HIV disease, will need on-site psychiatric services in order to maintain these challenging patients in the community and to decrease the need for psychiatric or medical hospitalization.

Mobile treatment units that meet patients where they live may be one option for the care of homeless. University- and community-based agencies must be encouraged. Pooling academic and front-line resources will result in better understanding of the HIV population needing care, treatment ideas that work effectively, and archaic perspectives that must be abandoned. Psychiatrists must fully engage in the effort to abolish the stigma associated with HIV/AIDS and mental illness. Working with other physicians, non-physician providers of mental health care, patients, and families, psychiatrists can provide a unique perspective on the biopsychosocial/spiritual aspects of HIV disease and impact the highly political process that determines health policy. Until the economic stigma surrounding HIV disease and mental illness is decreased, HIV/AIDS patients needing psychiatric care will suffer.

The practice of psychiatry in the setting of HIV/AIDS must be determined by local circumstances and not merely by ideology. The increasing complexity of mental illness in HIV-infected patients demands the best that all providers can offer. General psychiatric practice of the future, as well as HIV-specific psychiatric practice, demands better definition of diagnostic subtypes in order to achieve improved treatment outcomes. Is the depression seen in an AIDS patient due to a "major depressive episode" or to depression associated with AIDS dementia? Do the two illnesses respond equally well to current modes of depression therapy, or does a different etiology require a different intervention?

Improvement in diagnosis will also achieve more uniform application of diagnostic labels, resulting in better communication among care providers. Improvement in identification and communi-cation will then allow a clearer definition of treatment outcomes, providing the opportunity for a clearer demon-stration of benefit from psychiatric services. Future advances in the understanding of individual drug metabolism will facilitate more individualized dose-response targets for each patient. In other words, patients may one day benefit from truly individualized medication treatment plans, rather than population-based medication dosage recommendations. This is especially important in HIV/AIDS patients, who tend to be prescribed ten and twenty medications simultaneously, to be particularly susceptible to adverse medication effects, and to exhibit altered patterns of drug metabolism. Psychiatrists can serve many roles in the provision of care to HIV/AIDS patients, even when those patients receive the bulk of their care from other providers.

Psychopharmacology for AIDS

Many patients seek mental health care from a non-physician provider because medication is not their treatment of choice. Patients deserve to have clear explanations of the risks and benefits of medication for a given psychiatric illness in making this choice. It is important for non-physician providers of mental health care to HIV/AIDS patients to form a relationship with a psychiatrist purposes of medication consultation and referral, by taking these steps:

1) If possible, find a consultant with HIV/AIDS experience and interest. Medication management in HIV/AIDS patients is complex. Differentiating medication side effects from underlying illness or other possible causes requires special understanding of the biopsychosocial/spiritual aspects of HIV/AIDS.

2) Develop a relationship with the consultant before it is needed. It is always easier to call and ask a question of someone you know than it is to call someone "out of the blue." Be clear about your agenda in establishing a relationship with a consultant, and determine what the consultant sees as limitations to that relationship.

3) Remain neutral in your discussion with the patient about the "best" treatment options. As in any other area of the therapeutic relationship,

neutrality is vital. Allow exploration of issues such as whether to use medications or which particular medication is most appropriate. Help the individual to clarify his or her own biases without introducing your own.

4) If a referral for a medication evaluation is made, obtain releases of information, and provide the consul-tant with as much information about the individual's illness and potential need for medication as possible. Important information to include in your referral includes:

— Demographics, such as age, ethnicity, and relation-ship status.

— HIV disease status, including category (A,B,C), T-helper (CD_4) count/CD_4 per cetn/viral load (if known). If you do not know or feel comfortable about gathering this information, give the psychiatrist the name and the phone number of the patient's physician.

— Past psychiatric diagnoses, including substance use.

— Current psychiatric diagnoses, including substance use.

— Current symptoms that suggest a need for medication (*i.e.*, why you are making a referral).

— Past medication trials, if any, including the patient's experience with the medicine.

— Concerns the patient has expressed about seeing a psychiatrist or using medication.

In making a referral for a medication evaluation, it is important to be clear with the client and the consultant about the working relationships between each of you and how information will be shared after the consultation occurs.

In addition to helping to resolve psychopharmacology questions, psychiatrists can assist with diagnostic conundrums. HIV/AIDS patients may have several things going on simultaneously: mental illness, substance use, HIV-related illness, and other physical illness.

Obtaining a second opinion on a patient's condition can help clarify your treatment approach as well as reassure the patient, who may be concerned that symptoms represent the first stages of some frightening illness, such as dementia. A unique aspect of HIV/AIDS is the psychiatric presentation of many serious, and in some cases life-threatening, neurological diseases. In cases where a patient presents with psychiatric symptoms in the setting of severe immunocompromise (T-helper or CD_4 count less than 200: CD_4% less than 14), a psychiatric referral is indicated to ensure that a medical explanation for the symptoms cannot be found.

In cases where the person is mildly to moderately immunocompromised (CD_4 count between 200 and 500), a phone consultation is warranted to determine if farther evaluation is necessary. It is important to remember that any change in mental status, even a relatively subtle one that develops over a period of weeks, may reflect an underlying physical problem. It is best to err on the side of referral.

The nonphysician provider may be the first to encounter this change in the person and therefore has the responsibility of informing the patient's other providers if the patient cannot do this her or himself. With HIV disease, the borders between the biological, psychological, social, and spiritual disappear. Individual practitioners, regardless of their disciplines, need to acknowledge this and practice accordingly. Institutions and agencies can no longer retain divisive care systems when dealing with a condition that demands new, integrated models of care. HIV-1B is extremely rare in Africa, but a few strains have been found in certain countries of the sub-Saharan rain forest: Gabon, Cameroon, Ivory Coast, Uganda, and Rwanda. Proto-1B must have reached Europe from one of these areas, but probably not Uganda or Rwanda. Before 1940, the lack of commercial air transportation made these interior countries virtually inaccessible.

The virus more likely came by ship from a coastal area. It could have come from Ivory Coast, then a French colony, but since 1939 the epidemic began in Germany, a German colony is more logical. This points to Cameroon, which then included the northern parts of Gabon. Proto-1B must have descended from the African ancestor of all HIV-1 subtypes. Even if not always fatal, a serious disease would have been noticed in a colony like Cameroon, a colony with a good infrastructure dating back to the nineteenth century. Historical records would tell us if a deadly illness was endemic among colonists or local plantation workers. It would have made the country less prosperous and attractive to European superpowers, but England, France, and Germany never stopped fighting for this treasure. No reports hint that Cameroon was a dangerous place to colonize. So we can assume that, in colonial times, most HIV strains circulating in the territory must have been harmless and unnoticeable. They were largely unable to cause disease and, as will be argued, had not yet grown into subtypes.

The strain that became proto-1B had deadly potential but perhaps never caused *P. carinii* pneumonia (PCP) or other opportunistic infections and tumours until it got to Europe. This odd variant that mutated into a disease-causing virus no doubt left Cameroon by sheer chance. Proto-1B would have been closely related to the common HIV-1 ancestor, so that ancestor must have lived nearby. Whereas proto-1B ultimately went to Europe, other descendant strains travelled eastward in Africa. Like proto-1B, they would evolve from harmless to AIDS-causing viruses, mainly HIV-1A.. And if HIV subtypes form only during an epidemic in which disease is linked to passage among human hosts, then this same area gave rise to all the HIV-1 subtypes that favour heterosexual transmission.

Only HIV-1B, which favours homosexual transmission, developed its full potential elsewhere—in Europe. This historical scenario, with its two paths, may explain the divergence of 1B from the others: its preferential spread through anal intercourse versus their spread through vaginal intercourse. Since the common ancestor in Cameroon was harmless, a few HIV-1 strains could unknowingly be transported eastward, where they would quietly evolve by heterosexual passage. Likewise, strains that remained in Cameroon and Gabon evolved, unnoticed, into what became proto-1B. Then, during epidemics in Europe and the United States, they formed HIV-1B, the only HIV-1 subtype formed through serial passage by anal intercourse.

The common ancestor of HIV-1 must have passed from its source animal to humans in some outlying part of Cameroon, in the deep rain forest where people would be hunting and eating this animal. Once cross-species transmission had occurred, a human epidemic was perhaps inevitable.

Given enough time, the natural movements of African peoples might eventually have given HIV-1 the opportunity to become a large-scale human killer. But as it happened, the evolution of dangerous HIV-1 subtypes was vastly assisted by German colonialism. European colonialism caused turmoil in Africa, especially the mixing and movement of peoples.

Europeans not uncommonly had sexual relations with their subject people. In Cameroon, for example, many German officials reportedly had local black mistresses. These relationships sometimes erupted in scandal and bloodshed. We can assume that circulating HIV strains, though relatively harmless, were sometimes passed from Africans to Germans by sexual transmission.

In this same period there were major military movements against subject people who rebelled against cruelty and injustice. Such movements of the army and particularly the navy gave HIV ample opportunity to spread from one territory to another. It is easily envisioned that, around the turn of the century, a German sailor or adventurer-or an African servant-became infected in Cameroon and took the virus, by ship, to German East Africa, on the other side of the continent.

Most important, the Europeans used Africans in their colonial armies. The majority of soldiers on both sides of the African conflict were Africans. The colonial powers also recruited Africans to fight their battles in Europe. At the end of World War I, German colonies were distributed among the victors. In 1919 the Belgians claimed Rwanda and Burundi; the British took the rest of East Africa. The French took 80 per cent of Cameroon and Britain took 20 percent. By this time, HIV-1 was already seeded around Lake Victoria, where it would grow slowly into HIV-1A and the other African HIV-1 subtypes. But what about HIV-1B?

The first cases of opportunistic PCP and cytomegalovirus (CMV) infections and tumours did not occur in Germany until 1939. If German colonists coming home after World War I brought proto- 1B, we would expect such cases to occur in the 1920s. How do we account for the lag time? Apparently those returning expatriates were not infected, or else they carried harmless strains of HIV. The potentially lethal proto-1B must have been imported later among about three hundred Germans who came home in 1939 when war was declared between England and Germany.

9

Laws for AIDS Prevention and Education

Since HIV is most commonly transmitted through sexual intercourse or shared needles, explicit information is required about these activities—activities which are not openly discussed in many societies. Information is necessary, but in itself is not sufficient to bring about behavioural change.

HIV is transmitted primarily through behaviour which is private, secret, often hidden, and in many places illegal. Individual decisions and actions in the areas of sexuality and drug use do not necessarily follow the rules of logic or rationality however much we would like them to. They are areas of human behaviour which are subject to strong emotions and passions, often illogical and sometimes "dangerous".

The experience of HIV educators is that people need more than just information, even explicit information. Just as people continue to smoke even though the evidence of adverse health consequences is clear, people continue to engage in unsafe sex and needle sharing, even when they have full access to information about HIV transmission.

HIV educators face the following complex tasks:

— Provide explicit information about the virus and how it is spread.

— Provide explicit information about how individuals can protect themselves.

— Persuade the individual that HIV constitutes a real risk for him or her;

— Empower people to take action to protect themselves.

Information and education must be supplemented by other programmes, for example, ensuring that the blood supply is safe and that condoms and safe injecting equipment are readily available.

Information and education are also important to the second major aspect of HIV/AIDS programmes-minimizing the social and personal impact of HIV infection. People with HIV, or people who think they may be at risk of acquiring HIV, must not be frightened of presenting themselves for testing or treatment.

If people fear stigmatization or discrimination, they will be dissuaded from coming forward. This has implications not only for the health of the individual, but also for HIV prevention, as people who do not know their status are more likely to transmit the virus to others. Fear campaigns, or education campaigns which "demonize" people with HIV, can thus be counterproductive for people with HIV and society generally.

International laws

The International Covenant on Civil and Political Rights recognizes in Article 19 the right to information as a universal human right:

1. Everyone shall have the right to hold opinions without interference.
2. Everyone shall have the right to freedom of expression; this right shall include freedom to seek, receive and impart information and ideas of all kinds, regardless of frontiers, either orally, in writing or print, in the form of art, or through any other media of their choice.
3. The exercise of the rights provided for in paragraph 2 of this article carries with it special duties and responsibilities. It may, therefore, be subject to certain restrictions, but these shall only be such as are provided by law and are necessary:
    a) For respect of the rights or reputations of others,
    b) For the protection of national security or of public order (order public), or of public health or morals.

Also relevant to HIV/AIDS information and education are Article 21 (the right of peaceful assembly) and Article 22 (the right to freedom of association).

National laws

Most of the countries have laws, often contained in their Constitution or Bill of Rights, which assert general rights to information, freedom of expression, or freedom of speech. The Constitution of the Philippines explicitly provides for "the right of the people to information on matters of public concern", as well as ancillary rights of freedom of speech, freedom of expression, and freedom of the press.' In Papua New Guinea, section 46 of the Constitution guarantees freedom of expression, which is defined to include freedom to hold and communicate opinions and information, and specifically guarantees freedom of the press and mass media.' Article 19 (l) (a) of the Constitution of India guarantees the right to freedom of speech and expression to all persons.'

The enforceability of constitutional guarantees, varies between countries, depending on the structure of the Constitution and the legal system generally. However, such guarantees are invariably subject to exceptions, sometimes explicitly stated or implicit in judicial interpretation. Exceptions commonly relate to such issues as defamation, national security, morality or obscenity.

Article 19(2) of the Constitution of India qualifies the right to freedom of speech guaranteed in Article 19 (1), in making it subject to reasonable restrictions that may be imposed by law in the interests of the sovereignty and integrity of India, the security of the State, friendly relations with foreign States, public order, decency or morality, or in relation to contempt of court, defamation or incitement to an offence.

AIDS education programmes

The information on sexually trasnmitted diseaces may be conveyed in a variety of ways, including posters, printed pamphlets, performances, movies, videos, radio, television, telephone, computer games and networks, lectures, group discussions, and individual counselling. A wide range of different laws is likely to apply to these various situations. However, the law is only one among several factors that determine what can be portrayed or discussed in these various situations.

The content of AIDS information and education materials and programmes depends on a wide range of factors, starting with the nature of the target group. How is the target group at risk? What information do they need to change their behaviour? What is the best way of getting through to them? What is their level of literacy or general education? What will offend or shock them? Is it a good idea for people to be offended or shocked? Will this galvanize them into action or will it merely prompt them to switch off or ignore the message? Will the television station be prepared to telecast educational programmes? Will commercial advertisers object to "unpleasant" subjects being portrayed alongside the advertisements for their products? Who decides whether a film or video can be shown, and in particular whether it can be shown to children? Will printers object to printing the pamphlet? Will the school principal permit an open discussion? Will the local council allow the poster to be displayed? Will religious bodies support or oppose the proposed material or programme? Will funding bodies object? These are some of the complex questions that AIDS educators confront regularly, in addition to the potential problems posed by the law. Lawyers must look far and wide to identify the many different laws which impact HIV/AIDS prevention and education.

Depending on the political and legal system, such laws may be national, state or provincial, or local government laws. Religious and customary law is also significant in some countries.

The relevant laws and regulations existing in many countries include:

— Obscenity laws.

— Laws about advertising or promotion of condoms.

— Laws prohibiting advertisement of false cures or treatments.

— Laws regulating the licensing and content of television and radio.

— Laws regulating the classification, distribution and exhibition of films and videos.

— Laws regulating the printing and distribution of printed materials.

— Customs laws regulating the importation of films, videos and printed materials.

— Laws regulating advertising.

— Local government laws regulating aspects such as advertising in public transport, public toilets, or on billboards.

— Laws against promotion or assistance of criminalised activities.

— Laws about school education.

— Laws about prisons.

— Laws against vilification of certain social groups. Religious or customary laws.

— Laws affecting the status of women.

— Laws about the use of national or minority languages. Laws about dealing with or assisting illegal immigrants.

— Laws restricting the ability to form community-based organizations, either generally or for particular groups (e.g., sex workers, injecting drug users, homosexuals).

— Laws restricting the use of government funding.

— Government guidelines on the content of HIV education programmes.

Some of these laws are very prescriptive and clear; whereas many others are likely to give wide scope for administrative or judicial discretion. Several of these laws overlap with each other. Others tend to place restrictions on HIV/AIDS education and information; however, some of them may be used to overcome or challenge restrictions.

Obscenity laws

Most countries have laws prohibiting obscene or pornographic materials or actions. What is considered obscene varies considerably from one place to another, and from time to time, depending on the prevailing social and moral values.

As an example, Section 292 of the Indian Penal Code makes it an offence to sell, hire, distribute, exhibit and circulate obscene books, pamphlets, paper writings, drawings, paintings, representations, figures or any other objects. Exceptions are made if the publication is for scientific, literary or higher learning, or bona fide religious purposes, or if the material is sculpted, painted, depicted or represented on ancient monuments or temples.

Section 293 of the Code makes the sale of obscene products to young people punishable, and section 294 of the Code makes it an offence to commission an obscene act and/or sing or recite or utter an obscene song, ballad or words in or near a public place. In India, "obscene" is defined as that which is lascivious or appeals to the carnal interest or tends to deprave or corrupt those to whom it is addressed. This definition, as in most countries, is very subjective and open to a broad interpretation.

This particular provision came into the Indian Penal Code during British colonial rule, and similar provisions appear in the laws of many countries in this region. It is clear that such a view of obscenity has not always been a part of India's values—as demonstrated by the reference to ancient temple carvings, which explicitly portray a range of sexual couplings.

In the Malaysian Penal Code, that prosecution would be unlikely "if materials carrying information on HIV/AIDS are genuinely educational in nature". This comment confirms the wide discretion possessed by authorities in the area of obscenity.

When obscenity is assessed by a reference to "community standards", the question which arises is, which community? In every society there is likely to be a wide range of standards, and different communities are likely to be offended by different things. This is a real issue for HIV/AIDS educators, who need to target programmes at particular groups within society.

Are sex workers, for example, likely to be "depraved or corrupted" by exposure to sexually explicit language or depictions of sexual conduct? Gay men are not likely to be shocked or depraved by a depiction or discussion of homosexual conduct, whereas some non-homosexual people may be disgusted by any mention of homosexuality.

Young people are most at risk of contracting HIV. Should educational material targeted at them be judged by the standards of older people, who may be more conservative? Some religious leaders would argue that chastity and fidelity are the only ways to counter HIV/AIDS, and are opposed to condom use in any circumstances. They may contend that any suggestion of condom use, even in the context of HIV/AIDS, is likely to "deprave and corrupt".

Laws for promotion of condoms

One of the central part of of HIV prevention programmes is condom promotion. However, some countries have laws banning or restricting the advertisement or promotion of condoms. In many countries, though, such restrictions have never existed or have been removed to facilitate family planning and HIV/AIDS programmes. In Australia, for example, the state government of Victoria prohibited advertising of condoms under the Police Offences (Contraceptives) Act 1935. Apart from issues of morality or propriety, this law was supported by such "arguments" as that the "Australian race" would disappear if contraceptives were widely used, that young people should not be able to indulge themselves without any responsibility, and that wealthier (i.e., better) people were limiting the size of their families through condom use. Until recently, condoms could not be openly displayed or advertised in Australia. Since the onset of the HIV/ AIDS epidemic, laws and practices have changed radically, and condoms are now openly sold in such places as supermarkets and are advertised in the press, on television, and on the sides of buses.

In Myanmar, condoms were banned until 1992 and are still not widely available or promoted. In Cambodia, a 1992 survey by the Ministry of Public Health found that 77 per cent of the population said they did not know what a condom is or about its use in protecting against HIV/AIDS. In Vietnam, a man who hosted a "condom party", at a Ho Chi Minh City hotel, was jailed in 1993 for "degrading national culture." A year later it was reported that the HIV epidemic had led the Vietnamese government to break with the past, and officially sanctioned pamphlets had been issued warning: "If you don't have a condom, don't get drunk." In Malaysia, condom advertisements are not allowed in the electronic media, but are permitted in the print media with the proviso that the advertisements are in the context of HIV prevention. In Papua New Guinea, whilst there is no bar to condom with condom promotion as such, there have been problems packaging and instructions for use. In 1991 a line of condoms sold under the brand name "Protector" was marketed in Papua New Guinea, with an instruction insert in Pidgin, the national language. The condoms were a great success. But conservative Christian forces complained to the National Centralsorship Board, which found the insert to be pornographic because the line drawings implied the presence of a sexual partner while the man was putting the condom on. All stores selling the condoms were ordered to remove the inserts, until the drawings were altered to remove the visible legs of the "sexual partner".' A similar problem exists in Fiji with pictorial depictions of condom use in instruction inserts.

In Japan, on the other hand, legal and social barriers to condom promotion are minimal:

> .. distribution is widespread, supermarkets everywhere carry stocks, conveniently placed next to women's sanitary goods, as it is Japanese women who are the main condom buyers. Vending machines are also common, although there are initial problems with children mistaking them for bubblegum machines (which probably put a lot of Japanese children off bubblegum for life). In Japan, distribution is so widespread that women even sell condoms door-to-door. One brand was actually packaged to look like an encyclopedia.... Furthermore, packaging is as attractive and tempting as possible. Leading Japanese commercial artists are employed to promote condoms in the same way as any other household items; novelty packaging, accessories

and gimmicks are all part of the incentive to buy. You can buy condom packs disguised as cigarette boxes or as packs of cosmetics; some condoms even have musical movements activated when the packet is opened."

Laws prohibiting advertisement of false cures

False cures and treatment for HIV/AIDS is obviously counterproductive to HIV education. Such cures or treatment may be promoted simply as a moneymaking scam, or because of a genuinely misguided belief on the part of the promoter. In either case, gullible people may be persuaded to part with their money and put their health at risk.

In Papua New Guinea, section 140 of the Public Health Act makes it an offence to publish statements promoting the sale of any medicine, instrument or appliance for the alleviation or cure of venereal diseases, complaints or infirmities arising from or relating to sexual intercourse, diseases affecting generative functions, etc.

The provision does not apply to publications in relation to medical research, and publications sent to medical practitioners or pharmacists for the purpose of their businesses, or advertisements approved by the Commissioner for Venereal Diseases. Such a provision will appear in the laws of other countries. However, many people (including people with HIV/AIDS) have strong beliefs in traditional and herbal remedies. It is difficult for the law to strike a balance between the protection of people from fraud, and allowing for genuine belief in the efficacy of traditional and herbal remedies.

In Thailand, there was an uproar in early 1994 when the owner of Living with Nature Club in Chiang

Mai was arrested and charged with distributing herbal water without a license and defrauding the population. Over 1,000 people with HIV were members of the club. Angered by the arrest, a group of people with HIV protested. The group swore they were not victims of deception, and received support from non-governmental organizations. They sent representatives to see the Prime Minister, asking the government to reconsider its action and show compassion for the people depending on the man's herbal medicines to treat their condition. As a compromise, the Public Health Ministry allowed association members to continue preparing their herbal treatment.

Laws regulating content of television and radio

Many countries in the Asia-Pacific region exercise very tight control over radio and television broadcasting. Some exercise a government monopoly on broadcasting, not permitting any competition to government-owned stations. In other countries, there is a mix of government and commercial operators, with decision-making about content and censorship powers sometimes being delegated to the broadcasters themselves. Censorship (including self-censorship) of sexual content in the electronic media is stricter than for other forms of media because of its accessibility to all age groups throughout the region who have the necessary equipment.

At the same time, because of their extensive reach, television and radio are attractive and important for HIV/AIDS information and education campaigns. In Australia, where the attitudes towards sexuality are relatively liberal, the Department of Health has run several major AIDS campaigns on television.

However, television advertisements are the subject of self-regulation by a non-government body, the Federation of Australian Commercial Television Stations (FACTS), which the Department of Health regularly consults before launching its campaigns:

> "In 1989, following discussions with FACTS at the script development stage, the Department of Health decided not to accept a proposal to include homosexual couples in the 'Beds' television commercial, which had originally only been planned for heterosexual couples... FACTS had advised that it may have difficulty giving the advertisement clearance, and even if it did, some member stations would probably refuse to broadcast it. Some stations, such as the regional television station in North Queensland, declined to even screen the final version of the commercial showing heterosexual couples only.

An international AIDS journal has reported the following incident in Pakistan:

> "As a report about AIDS in Poland begins on BBC's Health File', the scrambler in Pakistan Television Corporation's control room rushes into action, distorting the picture and muffling the sound. It is almost a reflex action on the part of the official on duty because the government's censorship policies do not prohibit AIDS-related news or features. But the practice is common in many Muslim countries. 'If they are talking of AIDS, sex can't be far behind', says a TV official in Pakistan."

Media regulation laws are not only about censorship-they also have the capacity to be used to the advantage of HIV/ AIDS educators. For example, an expert committee in Australia has recommended that the government should require television and radio broadcasters to provide free time for community service announcements which would include HIV/AIDS and other government health promotion campaigns, and that announcements should be screened at a variety of times including prime time. The committee noted that the Australian Minister for Communications already had the power to direct broadcasters to broadcast information of "national interest", and that this should be broadened to include "community interests" enabling the Minister to direct that broadcasters carry information relating to serious threats to health, including HIV/AIDS.

Laws regulating film and video

Many countries have legally established systems for the censorship and classification of films and videos. Films are often censored or classified on the basis of sexual or violent content, and also for political reasons.

In India, before being exhibited, all films must have a certificate under the Cinematograph Act 1952. The Act states that a film shall not be certified if, in the opinion of the authority, the film or any part of it is against the interest of the sovereignty and integrity of India; the security of the state; friendly relations with foreign states; public order; decency or morality or involves defamation or contempt of court, or is likely to incite the commission of an offence. Guidelines have been framed by the central government, including a guideline stating that visuals or words depicting women in ignoble servility to man or glorifying such servility as a praiseworthy quality shall not be permitted.

Moreover, the authority is to ensure that the film is examined in the light of contemporary standards of the country and the people to which the film relates.

In Australia, films are generally classified by the Commonwealth Office of Film and Literature Classification. This office has stated that its general principles applied to film and video classification are as follows:

— Adults should be free to see what they wish provided there is sufficient protection for young people, and those people who do not wish to see certain material should not have it thrust upon them.

— The classification should reflect what a reasonable adult person would consider within the acceptable limits of community standards for that age group.

— The closest attention is paid to the portrayal of violence and, in particular, sexual violence.

— Certain classes of activity, such as sexual child abuse, bestiality, and the incitement to or encouragement of crime or violence are refused classification.

Laws regulating the printing materials

Some countries maintain a tight control over the publishing of newspapers and magazines by requiring licensing or registration, as well as monitoring content. Other countries allow a free press, but there are invariably a range of laws determining the content, and in some cases, how the publications may be distributed. In Australia, the office of Film and Literature Classification also classifies printed matter in most states and territories. It is a voluntary scheme; materials are only classified if they are presented for classification or if a complaint is lodged. They may be classified into one of four categories:

— Unrestricted

— Restricted Category 1 (restricted to persons over 18 years and must be displayed in a sealed wrapper).

— Restricted Category 2 (restricted to persons over 18 years of age and displayed for sale only in restricted premises).

— Refused Classification.

In Queensland, category 1 and category 2 material is banned, while other states operate their own classification systems. The Office has shown some flexibility in classifying HIV/ AIDS education material. For example, the Office was asked to classify a very explicit pamphlet "Six Tips for Hard Cocks", produced by the AIDS Council of NSW for gay men, demonstrating the proper use of condoms. The pamphlet was given an "Unrestricted" classification, based on an undertaking that it would be distributed to adults only in places such as gay bars. This was an important recognition of the need for explicit, targeted information in HIV/AIDS education, and of the fact that material which might be considered offensive to some parts of the community should be permitted distribution to targeted groups.

Laws regulating importation of films, videos and printed materials

The customs laws of countries often judge imported materials by criteria different from those applied to locally produced materials. This has implications for HIV/AIDS educators who wish to import AIDS materials from overseas. HIV/ AIDS educators often get ideas from each other, and use or emulate successful campaigns and materials from other countries.

At international conferences and study tours, information and materials are often exchanged. It is important that educators should not have to keep reinvesting the wheel. Educators returning to some home countries may have to bear in mind the possibility that their newly acquired material may be examined and possibly confiscated by the customs authorities, and that they may even be subject to prosecution for attempting to import sexually explicit material, or material which is explicit about injecting drug use. In Australia, the Customs (Prohibited Imports) Regulations apply to films, slides, video tapes, video discs and any other form of recording from which a visual image can be produced, books, papers, magazines, films or other written or pictorial matter. Regulation 4A (4) says that importation of the following goods is prohibited unless permission is obtained from the Attorney-General:

— Pictures of child pornography or of bestiality, likely to cause offence to a reasonable adult.

— Pictorial representation of acts of considerable violence or cruelty or of sexual violence against non-consenting persons.

— Publications and films that promote or incite crime, violence or drug abuse.

If films or videos are for public exhibition, they must first be registered. It can be seen that there is duplication and potential conflict with the domestic process for approval and classification.

Advertisement regulating laws

In Australia advertising is self-regulated by the media industry, where most decisions are made by an Advertising Standards Council. This body has often ruled against health promotion advertisements, including anti-smoking and HIV/AIDS campaigns, on the grounds of taste and decency. In September 1990 the Advertising Standards Council banned the Victorian AIDS Council's poster showing two men kissing with the headline 'When you say Yes, Say Yes to Safe Sex'. The ban came in response to a complaint by a coalition of church and community groups in Bendigo, who claimed that the advertisement breached several clauses of the Media Council Codes, including that it was misleading and deceptive and would cause serious offence to a significant section of the community.

Although the Council noted that it was the type of advocacy advertisement where it has traditionally allowed wide latitude to advertisers, it concluded that the material 'went way beyond the bounds of advocacy and acceptability to community Standards.' The Council said it appeared that the advertisement was 'less concerned with the prevention of AIDS and more concerned with encouraging homosexuality' and was likely to cause serious offence to a significant section of the community. One of the difficulties caused by such a system of self-regulation is that there is no right of appeal against such a decision.

Regulation of advertising in such places as public transport, public toilets or billboards is often the responsibility of local governments. Powers may be found in local government legislation or planning and environment legislation. There is the potential for local authorities to use this power to censor HIV/ AIDS information and education material. In the Australian state of New South Wales, the Local Government Act 1919, gives councils the power to regulate advertisements and structures used or to be used for the display of advertisements. This power has occasionally led to problems for HIV educators. In late 1991, problems arose for the AIDS Council of NSW and the Wollongong and Shellharbour Council over the wording of a stencil to be used in council toilets as part of a 'Beat' programme. The original stencil said: 'Always use a condom when having anal or vaginal sex.' The Councils objected to the explicitness of the message and asked that it be replaced with 'Always use a condom When having casual sex'. Wollongong Council eventually agreed to use the stencil in its original form, but Shellharbour Council has refused to use it. In the Australian context, it has been recommended that local councils should not use their legislative powers to impede HIV-related health promotion campaigns.

In the United States, the Massachusetts Bay Transportation Authority refused in 1993 to place condom advertisements in its trolleys and subways. The advertisements, prepared by the AIDS Action Committee of Massachusetts, displayed a large colour picture of a condom wrapped in a package and messages stating that condoms are an effective means of preventing the transmission of HIV.

The advertisements used humour and suggestive language to overcome adolescents' and men's reluctance to use condoms. The AIDS Action Committee successfully sued, claiming violation of the First Amendment (freedom of speech) and the Fourteenth Amendment (due process) of the US Constitution.

The US District Court, upheld on appeal by the US 1st Circuit Court of Appeals, found in favour of the AIDS Action Committee. The court pointed out that at the same time as the Authority was refusing to run the condom ads, it was displaying sexually suggestive posters for a Hollywood movie featuring the bare, crossed legs of a woman. The court said that if the Authority was displaying commercial ads which were overtly sexual, it could not block public service ads of a more modest nature without running a foul of the First Amendment protection of freedom of speech. The court added that both sets of ads "fall well within the heartland of speech that we, as a secure society, should be willing to tolerate in the marketplace of ideas." It is inappropriate for local authorities to impede HIV/AIDS programmes designed and promoted at a national or state level. It must be remembered, though, that attitudes among local authorities vary enormously, and that local authorities may be able to use their powers to the benefit of HIV/AIDS programmes, even if there is indifference or hostility to such programmes at higher levels of government.

Laws for promotion of criminalised activities

In China, the National People's Congress passed a resolution in 1990 that a penal sentence is to be given to those who cajole, abet, deceive and/or coerce others to take or inject narcotic drugs. 12 One approach to HIV education with injecting drug users is to say that the only way to protect yourself against HIV is to stop using drugs. This is a method which has demonstrably failed, and has led to high rates of HIV infection amongst injecting drug users in places where it has been the sole strategy. In order to minimize infection, there is a need to be realistic and to say, in effect we accept that you are going to use drugs and this is how to do it safely. Such a message is not, in terms of the Chinese law, cajoling, deceiving or coercing, but it may be seen as abetting or assisting. Similar questions arise in other areas of HIV/AIDS education:

— If prostitution is illegal, is it lawful to talk to sex workers about strategies and sexual practices which aim to assist them in protecting themselves or their clients from HIV infection? Is this aiding or abetting acts of prostitution?

— If homosexual acts are illegal, is it lawful to talk about how to do them safely? Can programmes specifically targeted at gay men be seen as promoting homosexuality?

— Is it lawful to talk to young people below the age of consent about specific sexual practices?

Laws for sex education in schools

The school system is a crucial point for children and young people to be exposed to information about HIV/AIDS and how to protect themselves. Sex education has long been a controversial issue in most countries, and HIV/AIDS gives added urgency to the resolution of this issue. In the Philippines, a strong Catholic nation, debate has taken place in the legislature on the question of HIV education in schools.

Some legislation has supported the need for HIV education. However legislative counter reactions can also be seen in Senate Resolution No 314 which, while recognizing the necessity of teaching HIV prevention and control and integrating it into the high school curriculum, opposes the [Department of Education Culture and Sports] programmes of integrating into the First and Second Year High School's 'Physical Education, Health and Music' Programme the promotion and use of condoms, on the ground that such plans promote promiscuity among teenagers who should be taught moral values and standards instead. In the American state of Alabama, a bill was passed by the legislature in 1992 which stipulates that any sex education programme in Alabama public schools should include:

— That abstinence from sexual intercourse is the only completely effective protection against pregnancy and STDs, including AIDS when transmitted sexually.

— An emphasis on the importance of self-control and ethical conduct pertaining to sexual behaviour.

— An emphasis in a factual manner and from a public health perspective, that homosexuality is not a lifestyle acceptable to the general public and that homosexual conduct is a criminal offence under the laws of the state.

A familiar argument in this context is that sex education will increase sexual activity and might thus contribute to the transmission of HIV.

Michael Merson, formerly Executive Director of the World Health Organization's Global Programme on AIDS, argues the contrary view:

> "Research has shown that, contrary to popular belief, children who receive sex education do not become sexually active earlier than others. Quite the opposite: such youngsters delay their sexual experimentation, and when they do engage in intercourse they are more likely to take the right precautions, including contraception.

In many countries where there is extensive sex education and HIV education in schools, it remains a matter of dispute whether condoms should be promoted or made available in schools. For example, there has been extensive litigation on this issue in New York City.

In Thailand, the longtime condom promoter (and former Cabinet Minister) Mechai Viravaidya has no doubts about what is needed in school education:

> "Condom Man was last seen valiantly striding from bar to bar in Bangkok, talking with bar girls and patrons alike, always making surė to distribute his trusty condoms. Our plan... is to take Condom Man beyond the bars and have him reach a broader base. In fact, we plan to send him to where his popularity will be the highest and most effective: to school-age children. We have yet to secure the permission of the Thai Ministry of Education for this somewhat radical departure from traditional education, but I am confident that when Condom Man himself lands in the Minister's office, permission will be granted.

Prison laws

Prisons are environments which are potential hothouses of HIV transmission, because of the high level of injecting drug use, and the high level of sexual activity between men, both consensual and nonconsensual. HIV infection is not contained within the prison; prisoners are eventually released, and return to their families and regular lives, which may lead to further infections in the community.

Prison laws and regulations must provide for HIV education and information, and provide prisoners with the means to protect themselves from the virus. Prisons present a very clear example of the near futility of providing information and education without giving access to condoms and safe injecting equipment.

Laws for vilification of certain social groups

Stigmatization or discrimination against people with HIV/AIDS or affected communities will be counter productive for HIV information and education programmes. Bearing this fact in mind, the Australian state of New South Wales has passed laws against the vilification of people on the basis of their race, their sexual preference, or the fact that they have, or are thought to have, HIV. Under Section 49ZXB of the state's Anti-Discrimination Act.

> It is unlawful for a person, by a public act, to incite hatred towards, serious contempt for, or severe ridicule of a person or group of persons on the ground that the person is or members of the group are HIV/AIDS infected or thought to be HIV/AIDS infected.

The Act also creates a criminal offence of "serious HIV/ AIDS vilification", where the above acts occur by means which include:

— Threatening serious harm towards, or towards any property of the person or group of persons.

— Inciting others to threaten physical harm towards, or towards any property of, the person or group of persons.

The offence is punishable by a tine of up to $5,000 or imprisonment for six months or both.

Religious or customary laws

Some countries recognize religious or customary laws alongside their formal legal system. A good example of the impact these laws can have on HIV education programmes comes from Papua New Guinea:

> "As part of the public awareness campaign already instituted in the country, a man living with HIV from the Highlands area volunteered his services in various outreach programmes. He did an excellent job, travelling around villages all over the remote and rugged

> Highlands area, explaining, demonstrating, counselling. A video was made in which he starred in his role as an outreach worker. Shortly afterwards he died. The video has had to be suppressed. The subject is dead, and a dead person has passed into the spirit world and it is vital that his privacy be respected. If the video were to be released for public showing, his angry relatives would object and ask for compensation for the infringement of sacred taboos.

In some aboriginal communities in Australia, tribal elders have banned photos of male and female genitalia showing STD symptoms, even for same-sex audiences.

In Malaysia, the Islamic Syariah Law applies to Muslims. As premarital sex is prohibited under Islamic law, condoms cannot be given to unmarried persons in any official programmme, since this would suggest that the authorities are condoning premarital sex. Much of the content of HIV/AIDS, educational and information programmes is not, of course, customary in most cultures.

The advent of HIV/AIDS has meant that customs and cultures have had to change and adapt in order to minimize the harm to their communities. This is not to argue against the need for cultural appropriateness, or to doubt the validity of customary or religious laws. However, if the effect of customary law is to set customs in concrete or to create a perception that customary laws are unchangeable, this create problems for HIV/AIDS programmes. HIV/AIDS educators need to bear in mind that all cultures evolve and chance over time; none are static.

In Uganda, health workers believed that it was wrong to tell people that they have HIV because it is not customary to talk about death, dying or related issues. Despite this, a Ugandan NGO conducted surveys that found that people actually wanted to know if they were positive or negative, and they are now mobilizing support services and informing people of their HIV status, despite the supposed cultural inappropriateness.

Laws for women's status

Women are likely to be more difficult to reach with HIV/AIDS information and education programmes because of the laws and customs which subordinate and disempower them. Most of the countries treating women are the subordinate sex, relegated to second-class status, kept uneducated, dependent, isolated and confined within the four walls of their homes. They are often denied access to education, health, independent income and property rights. All these factors combine to increase women's vulnerability and obstruct any effective prevention campaign.

Laws for the use of languages

In some countries there are laws or legal systems which require the use of national languages in certain contexts and restrict the use of minority languages. Such legal requirements pose a number of problems for AIDS educators in reaching minority, indigenous populations, since material dealing with such sensitive and personal issues as sexual behaviour and drug use is often best presented in everyday, colloquial language. If HIV/AIDS education material is only presented in a language other than the person's mother tongue, the problems are:

— The material does not reach people who are not

literate or fluent in the official language.

— Even if people understand the words, will they understand the message?

— There may be a tendency for minority groups to see HIV as not applicable to them if it is not in their own language. It may be seen as a disease of the national majority group, rather than their own minority group.

These considerations apply not only to indigenous minorities, but also to immigrants. With uneven economic development, there is a huge influx of immigrant workers from one country to another country, often working in lowly paid jobs, poorly educated or illiterate even in their own languages.

In Malaysia, for example' there are over 1 million migrant workers in a population of 18 million, many of them from the neighbouring countries of Thailand and Indonesia. Article 26 (equality before the law) and Article 27 (rights of ethnic, religious and linguistic minorities) of the International Covenant on Civil and Political Rights have particular relevance to these situations. Many countries in the Asia-Pacific region have within them a wide variety of spoken and written languages. Reaching all these people is enough of a challenge to HIV/AIDS educators, without the additional burden of legal or bureaucratic restrictions on use of languages.

Laws to dealing with illegal immigrants

In many parts of the Asia-Pacific region there are large illegal population movements from country to country, caused by wars, political repression or instability economic opportunities, and other factors. Under the laws of most countries it is illegal to assist or harbour illegal immigrants.

In Thailand, for instance, large numbers of women and girls are recruited from neighbouring countries to the Thai sex industry. Many of these illegal immigrants come from rural farming communities and have little education, and little or no knowledge of HIV/AIDS. There is an obvious and pressing need for materials about HIV Written in different languages. The problem for non-government organizations is that if they work with illegal immigrants, they are likely to be breaking the law. In every country, illegal immigrants try to remain invisible; they do not wish to identify themselves for fear of arrest and deportation. While identifying them poses a major problem, HIV educators, do not, however, need the additional challenge of fearing arrest themselves merely for trying to work with these most marginalised communities.

Laws restricting the ability to create community based organizations

Whilst governments have a vitally important role in the fight against HIV/AIDS, community-based organizations also have a central role to play. Governments cannot do everything. They are subject to financial and logistical constraints. But more significantly, governments cannot hope to muster the same commitment or recognition or support as a community-based organization fighting to protect its own community. In Australia/ North America and parts of Europe, where the impact of HIV initially fell largely on gay men, organizations formed by the gay communities took much of the responsibility for responding to the epidemic.

The same phenomenon was observed in developing countries as diverse as Mexico, Zambia and Thailand. These organizations were able to formulate strategies to inform and educate their own communities in a way which governments either could not or were unwilling to do so. It is now recognized that the best way to reach injecting drug users is to empower organizations of injecting drug users to do so, and the most effective way of speaking to sex workers is to utilize sex worker organizations. The same principle applies to other groups and communities: both communities of interest and geographical communities. Women's organizations, youth groups, and organizations of ethnic and linguistic minorities, all have a role to play. Large-scale information campaigns, such as those run by governments, must be supplemented by peer education programmes which are more accessible to the individual. This principle was recognized in the 1986 Ottawa Charter for Health Promotion, which states that:

> "Health promotion works through concrete and effective community action in setting priorities, making decisions' planning strategies and implementing them to achieve better health. At the heart of this process is the empowerment of communities, their ownership and control of their own endeavours and destinies."

Rights of peaceful assembly and freedom of association are human rights recognized in the International Covenant on Civil and Political Rights. Despite this, some countries have laws which restrict the rights of people to organize themselves into groups. In some authoritarian countries there is a general prohibition on non-government organizations. In other countries there are considerable deterrents. Dennis Altman observes: "Knowing that one requires government registration to establish a group is a powerful deterrent from organizing, say, a sex workers' association in Indonesia or even a 'general' AIDS organization in Kuwait.""

Laws restricting the use of funds

NGOs working on HIV/AIDS education often rely on funding from governments, and this often comes with strict conditions on what it can be used for. Often, if a government is funding a non-government organization to produce educational material, the government reserves the right of final approval of the material, and also maintains copyright over material produced.

Material produced using government funding is more susceptible to protest from conservative elements of society than is material produced using money from other sources For example, a Safe Sex Diary produced by the Family Planning Association using Australian government funding had to be withdrawn from distribution after the Prime Minister had his attention drawn to it by a State Premier. This was not done through any formal legal process of censorship, but through the power of the government as the funding body, pursuant to the funding conditions.

Similar restrictions may be imposed by other organizations providing funding, such as development aid agencies or religious bodies.

Guidelines for HIV/AIDS programmes

Many governments have issued "guidelines" on the content of HIV/AIDS programmes. Guidelines might include standardised messages, with the rationale of ensuring consistency, avoiding counterproductive messages and avoiding the use of terms which may be considered as inappropriate or offensive. Whilst there may be benefits in standardized messages, this may become problematic if the guidelines do not allow messages to be tailored to particular target groups in terms the target groups can understand. There is, of course, potential for "guidelines" to be used as a defacto form of censorship, but this will not necessarily be the case if they are sufficiently flexib!e. Many of these laws predate the HIV-epidemic but eventhose laws which have been implemented or amended since the onsel of HIV are likely to have been made with no thought as to the consequences fo rHIV education.

Index